Endorsements

Love and wisdom emanate at the turn of each page. Maria's sincere desire to share both her experiences and research is captivating and encouraging! I felt confident that I too could have a healthy pregnancy at the end of each chapter. This is a must-read for any woman considering childbirth!

Vanessa, 4 months pregnant and mom of a toddler, Miami, FL

Maria combines the knowledge she gained from her personal birth experiences and her highly organized research skills to create *The Secrets to a Healthy Pregnancy*. She shares safe, practical knowledge while giving women confidence in their decision-making process and the courage to trust their bodies to birth their babies. Maria answers questions that parents have and explains options for many choices that modern couples don't even realize they have the right to make.

Sharain Santalla, Doula and Child Birth Mentor, Miami, FL

Maria caught my attention and drew me in from the very beginning. As a woman and mother who gave birth to four daughters at home (two through water births), I applaud Maria for recapturing these moments that are so very precious and memorable. I must admit that I was brought to tears in some parts as I recalled moments from my own experiences while reading this book. It's nice to know that there's an easy-to-read book with so much information for expectant parents. Readers will have a feel as to the true miracle of birth and realize that a natural home birth is an option if they choose.

Karen, married to Dr. Bartell, Deerfield Beach, FL

The Secrets To A Healthy Pregnancy

The Secrets To A Healthy Pregnancy

How to prepare to conceive, have a healthy pregnancy and childbirth, breastfeed successfully, and look HOT during it all!

Written by **Maria Wizel**

Illustrated by Romina Perez

Photography by:
Chris Sosa Photography
Alex Herrera Photography
GMN Artistic

Edited by:
Wendy Sola
Kelly Hall
Ceci Bonachea

LUCIDBOOKS

This book is based on my life-long journey to true health, two healthy pregnancies, my experience helping pregnant women, and extensive research in the area of health and wellness. I am not a medical professional. Consult one during your pregnancy. My goal is to coach you and prepare you mentally, emotionally, spiritually, and physically for the most intense 40 weeks of your life so that you can have your best possible pregnancy, a healthy baby, an amazing birth, and ultimately a healthier family.

This book is dedicated to my Lord, Jesus Christ
for blessing me with everything I have and everything I've lived.

And, to my grandmother, Andrea.
We were not able to cure you, but you inspired me to help others.
Te amo.

THE SECRETS TO A HEALTHY PREGNANCY
Copyright © 2014 by Maria Wizel

Illustrations by Romina Perez
Photography provided by Chris Sosa Photography, Alex Herrera Photography, and GMN Artistic.
Edited by Wendy Sola, Kelly Hall, and Ceci Bonachea

Published by Lucid Books in Houston, TX.
www.LucidBooks.net

All rights reserved. No part of this publication may be reproduced, stored in a retrieval system, or transmitted in any form by any means, electronic, mechanical, photocopy, recording, or otherwise, without the prior permission of the publisher, except as provided for by USA copyright law.

ISBN-10: 1632960109
ISBN-13: 978-1-63296-010-8

Special Sales: Most Lucid Books titles are available in special quantity discounts. Custom imprinting or excerpting can also be done to fit special needs. Contact Lucid Books at info@lucidbooks.net.

Contents

Endorsements i

Foreword xi

Journey Toward True Health xiii

Acknowledgements xv

How the Two of Us Delivered Mila xix

Chapter 1   Preheating the Oven 1

Chapter 2   The Hall Pass Myth 17

Chapter 3   True Nutrition 21

Chapter 4   Working Out: From Burpees to Burp-ups 37

Chapter 5   Napping Isn't Just for Babies 45

Chapter 6   Naturopathic Treatment: The Natural Path 55

Chapter 7   How Chiropractic Changed My Life 67

Chapter 8   Enjoying Pregnancy 79

                Part One: Me Time 80

                Part Two: Bonding with Your Baby 85

                Part Three: Changes By Trimester 86

                Part Four: Let's Talk About Sex 89

Chapter 9	Winning the War Against Stress	93
Chapter 10	Preparing to Breastfeed Successfully	103
Chapter 11	Delivering Your Baby	117
	Part One: Labor	117
	Part Two: Creating the Right Birth Plan	124
	Part Three: Comparing Your Options	142
Chapter 12	Where Did My Body Go? Bouncing Back Post-Pregnancy	147
Chapter 13	Pain-Free Delivery	155
Bonus	Healthy Babies	165
Epilogue: Perspective of a Skeptical Husband		177
About the Author		179
Endnotes		181
Index		201
Photo Credits		207

Foreword

Maria's pregnancies were filled with wonder and delight! She questioned and wondered about all the tests, screenings, and procedures. She was delighted to learn the truth behind much of the overtesting and unnecessary procedures and was eager to try new alternatives. She marveled at the true simplicity and beauty of her pregnancies, labors, and births! She took her pregnancies by the reins and experienced the end results firsthand—two natural and healthy pregnancies. She looked forward to labor and birth with ease, anticipation, and excitement.

I have watched Maria's process in writing this book. First, she became pregnant with the desire to share what she experienced and discovered during her journey through childbirth. Now, she gives birth, and her labor of love produced this beautiful book—The Secrets to a Healthy Pregnancy!

It has been an honor to share these journeys with Maria. This book provides the reader with practical, simple, and helpful ways to achieve a healthy pregnancy and a natural birth with the added benefit of Maria's beautiful storytelling. Enjoy!

Sheila Simms Watson, LM, CPM
Licensed Midwife, Certified Professional Midwife

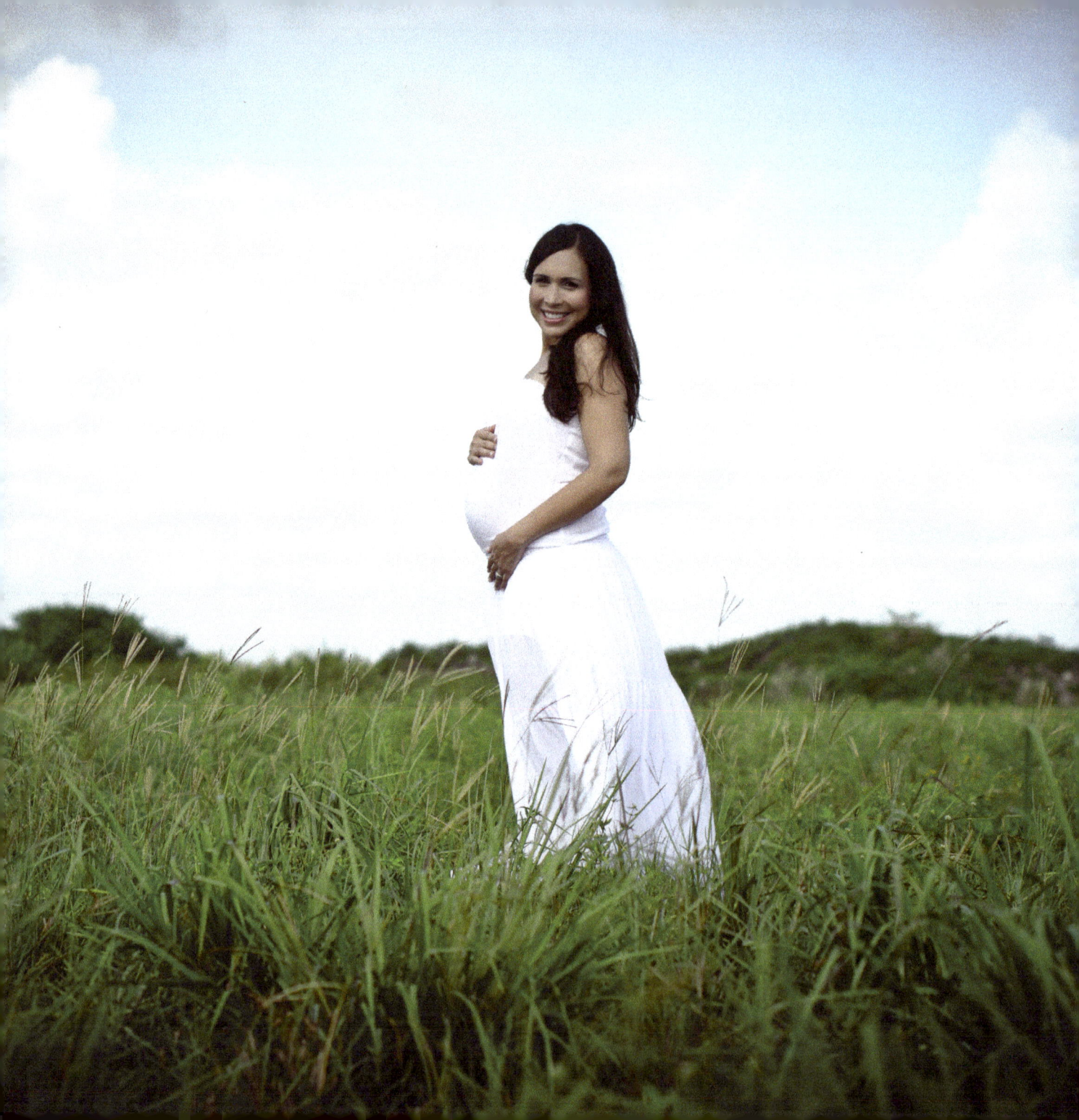

Journey Toward True Health

I wasn't always healthy; as a matter a fact, I was very sick. I was diagnosed with asthma when I was three. I remember being in and out of the hospital during my early childhood and seeing my mother and grandparents in agony because **I just couldn't breathe**. I continued to struggle with episodes of acute asthma during my teenage years and into adulthood, despite being under the care of great physicians, which included a pediatrician, an allergist, and a lung specialist—each one with a personal interest in me and giving me the best available care and prescriptions.

I was also overweight. I was a "chubby" kid growing up and a teenager with self-esteem issues because of my weight. This is when my mom placed me on naturopathic treatment and I became a vegetarian at 15. I was on a vegan diet for about one year and saw a big improvement in my overall health and weight. However, I lost my ways over time. Although I remained a vegetarian, my lifestyle was not healthy and my weight fluctuated like a yo-yo.

My grandmother was a respected registered nurse and college professor in our native Puerto Rico. She was always well-informed about medicine and common health practices. She, along with my grandfather and grandaunt, faithfully attended their array of doctors and took their prescription drugs as ordered. They were all under the best conventional medical care. They spent thousands of dollars on it (especially during their last years), but all of them lacked true health.

I lost my grandfather, grandaunt, and other members of my family to illnesses like cancer and diabetes when I was in my twenties. My grandmother fought Alzheimer's for over

a decade. The disease took hold of her body causing her to become bedridden even though she had the best conventional care.

I began learning about alternative medicine, eliminating toxic foods and going against the status quo during that time. I learned about how alternative medicine and a truly healthy lifestyle could help my grandmother, and I was hopeful for her. My mom and I were determined to help her get better. I even hoped to cure her. And this is why we zealously began our journey toward true health.

In 2011, I became pregnant with my first-born daughter, Bella. I was enjoying pregnancy until my asthma resurfaced around the third month. So, I sought the care of a naturopath. Not only did my asthma go away (once again), but she also encouraged and empowered me to consider a natural birth. She helped me throughout my entire pregnancy and beyond. I also began chiropractic treatment around that same time in an effort to treat a herniated disc that was becoming more and more bothersome as Bella grew in my womb. My chiropractors not only treated my back pain, but also taught me about true health and wellness. They supported my desire for a natural birth and helped me more than I thought a healthcare professional ever would.

Unfortunately, I lost my grandmother in 2012. Although our journey to her cure ended before we reached the goal, I learned so much along the way.

Life has a funny way of working things out. It was never about me, but I found true health throughout the process. What I learned became the foundation for my two healthy pregnancies and the reason I wrote this book. I have shared what I learned with my family, friends, and just about anyone who will allow me to. And now I want to share it with you. Knowledge is power. And I believe this book has the power to improve your health, so you can have a healthy pregnancy, baby, and birth.

I am honored and excited to embark on this journey with you. I hope you enjoy the ride!

Maria Wizel
November 9, 2014

Acknowledgements

Thank you:

To my husband, JC, for your love and support in making our book happen. It's the best ten year anniversary present I could have ever imagined.

To my four kids: Abi for sharing our stories, for your support, for helping me with the focus group and the amazing chapter titles. To John for sharing our stories so freely so that we can help others. Thank you Bella for your patience when I wrote during times we could have been playing. Thank you Mila for allowing me to breastfeed while writing. They were only babies when I started writing this book, but I knew it was important to share our stories while they were still fresh. I have the best children a mom could ever wish for.

To my mother, Ivonne, for being the best coach and role model. I treasure your advice with all of my heart. Your contributions to our book made it better. Thank you for being my #1 fan.

To Chris Sosa Photography for supporting me with great pictures from our early stages until the end. Thank you to Ginelle Lago at GMN Artistic for your gift of our beautiful group shot and my professional portrait. Thanks to Alex Herrera Photography for my pregnancy pictures and Bella's newborn photo. We never imagined they would end up in a book when we took them.

To my talented cousin and illustrator Romina, for the beautiful illustrations. I loved working with you. Your patience with me in the process is admirable.

To my mother in law, Doris, for lovingly supporting all my ways. Thank you for caring for me as your daughter.

To my dear friend, Ana, for watching, caring, and loving for my babies so that I could write.

To Sheila, for being the most amazing midwife I know, contributing in the labor chapter, and for writing the foreword.

To Dr. Gisela Fernandez at Healthy by Nature, for making me healthier, believing in our book, and for your contributions to the naturopathic care chapter.

To my chiropractors at Vivify Miami. To Dr. Lisa, for her relentless passion and dedication to her patients' health. To Dr. Joe, for reviewing and editing the chapter on chiropractic, and for educating us every chance he gets.

To my Puerto Rican, Mexican, and Guatemalan family for their love and support no mater the distance. Each of you is in this book through your influence in my life.

To Chelsey, Melissa, Jasmine, and Michelle for contributing with your ideas for the chapter titles. Thank you to all the girls who participated in our focus group.

To my friends and supporters of my blog and Facebook page for letting me be a part of your story, accepting my help, and sharing my posts with others.

To Pastor Bob for believing in me, encouraging me to write this book, and for your advice along the way. Thank you to his wife, Carey, for your love, openness, and willingness to share everything you know.

To Pastor Mark for your advice and your ideas for the title and subtitle. Thank you to his wife, Leilani, for sharing your beautiful conception story.

To Pastor John and Carolina for sharing Charlottes' beautiful birth story.

To my friends Evelyn, Samantha C., and Samantha L., you girls have been incredibly helpful in every step of this process, from sharing your stories, to your valuable feedback on my book and articles. I am blessed to have you as friends.

To the Matos Family for allowing me to share how their lifestyle and pregnancy stories impacted me on my journey to true health.

To Cecilia for allowing me to share your conception story and connecting me with your daughter Cecilia Maria Bonachea, my youngest editor. Ceci, you have been a blessing during this process.

To the rest of my editorial team: my friend Wendy Sola, you have been instrumental in this process. You joined my team in the very early stage of our book. I can't imagine this journey without you. And to the lovely and generous Kelly Hall, who began as an editor and is now a friend.

To Ivan "Ill Factor" Corraliza for recording the audio book.

To Casey and Marissa at Lucid books for believing in my book and helping my vision become a reality.

To Jesus Christ, my Lord and Savior. This book is for you. I wish my grandparents and grand aunt could have seen me become a published author. I know they would have been so proud. I know they are in your presence. And I have the certainty that I will see them again because of your love and sacrifice.

I love you all and thank you from the bottom of my heart.

MARIA

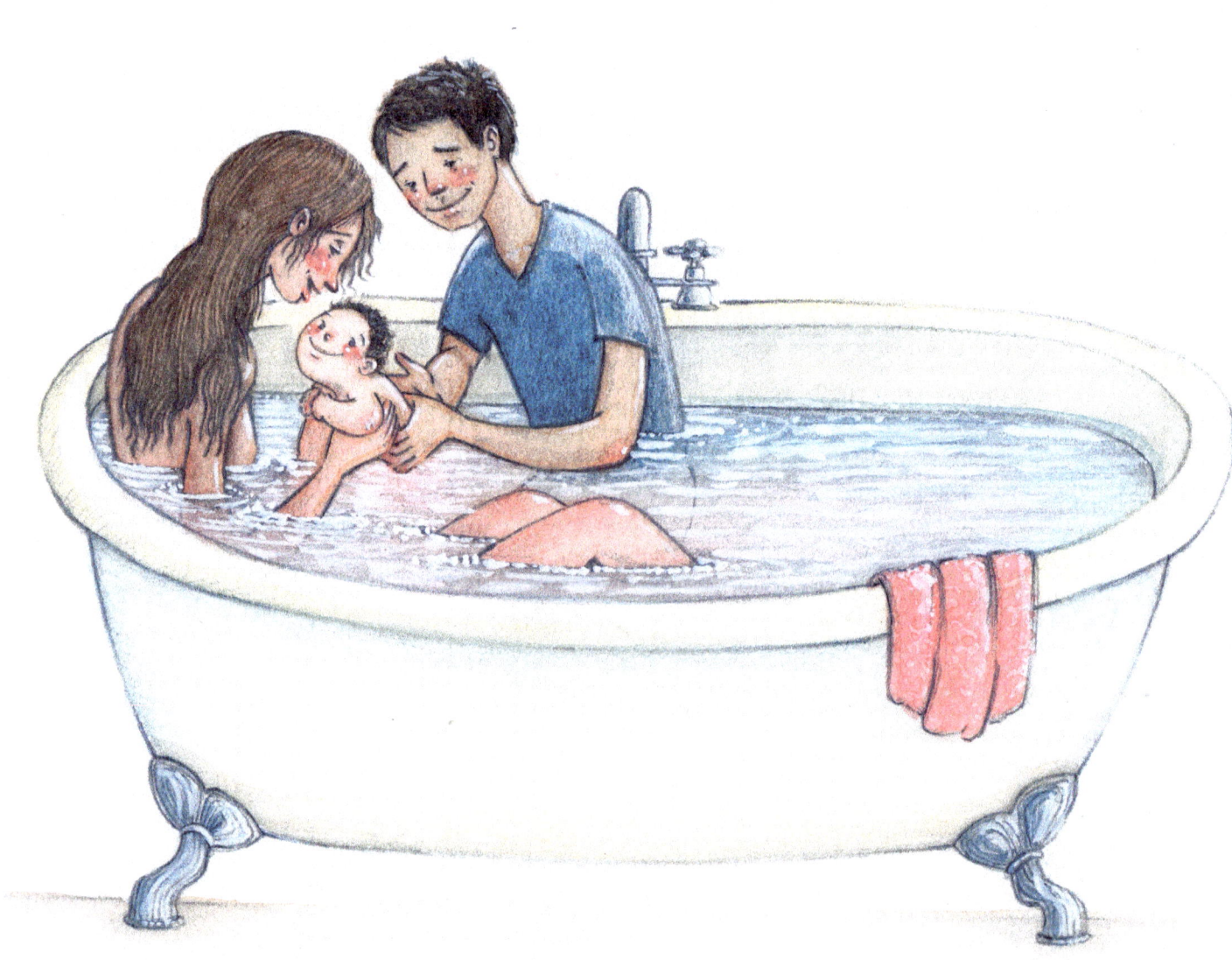

How the Two of Us Delivered Mila

Even when Bella was 22 months old, people were still asking me to tell the story about our beautiful home birth experience. My labor and delivery with Bella lasted 6 hours from the moment my water broke to the moment she was born. She was delivered in our bathtub surrounded by her father, both of her grandmothers, her big sister, and big brother. When I reached 39 weeks during my second pregnancy, I asked my midwife if I could expect Mila's birth to be faster than Bella's. She explained that each birth is unique, but that a good estimate would be half the time of Bella's birth—3 hours.

That day, I was three days short of 40 weeks. It was 3 AM, and I was an hour and a half into contractions. Everyone in my house was sleeping. I was free to walk around without anyone watching me and enjoy a soothing worship song on repeat titled Breathe[1]. My focus during my contractions was on my breathing. I was certain that Mila would be born that day. Unlike the Braxton-Hicks (or practice contractions) surfacing earlier that week, these contractions felt different. *They came with heat.*

My contractions were now closer together, and I felt like there was no longer a break between them. I decided it was time to wake up my husband, JC, and ask him to call Sheila, my midwife. After updating Sheila, he went to the bathroom and filled our tub with warm water in case I wanted to relax in there, but it felt better to stand up, so I went in the shower instead and let the cascading warm water relieve me.

Then, the baby descended unexpectedly and I knew that I couldn't stop her. I called for JC repeatedly to give him the news, "She's coming! She's coming!" I felt like she was going to fall out, so I put my right hand under me as if to sustain her and stretched out my left hand so that JC could help me get over to the bathtub, which was about seven feet away. "She's coming, babe!" I said with disbelief and excitement. He eased me into the bathtub and quickly called Sheila who said she was still about 20 minutes away. I could hear Sheila on the speakerphone. She asked a series of questions to make sure that we were safe.

I knew that Sheila wouldn't make it on time because I could feel Mila's head and couldn't resist the urge to push. Even with all the excitement, I felt confident in our ability to do it on our own. I could also sense JC's confidence and peace as he rose to the occasion. Mila's head came out with one long push. I took a few breaths and delivered the rest of her seven pound, nine ounce body. JC received Mila in the water and immediately put her on my chest. He checked to see that Mila was okay, and per Sheila's instruction, reached for a clean towel, soaked it in the warm water, and put it over Mila's back to keep us warm.

I will never forget the look on my husband's face! I looked into his eyes and admired how he delivered our baby with such courage. He praised me for birthing our baby, and we showered loving words upon one another. JC and I delivered our baby in a couple of minutes, just like that! Just the two of us alone in our bathtub, and then we were three! It couldn't have been any more beautiful.

I had been preparing for this day for months. I wanted labor to be as quick and easy as possible, but I never imagined it would be that fast and instinctive. I didn't plan it this way, but I surrendered to my body's natural course, and it turned out better than I had imagined.

I believe that the fulfillment of your birth plan begins with a healthy pregnancy. And preparing your body for pregnancy is the most important part of it. Making sure I was ready before conceiving was one of the wisest decisions I have ever made. Pregnancy can be tough! It takes a toll on you—physically, emotionally, and even psychologically! But as tough as it can be, I have never heard a woman say she wished she could go straight to holding her baby and skip pregnancy and labor. As women, we recognize that there is so much beauty in the process even though it is tough.

I liken pregnancy to a marathon, and skipping it would be like getting a medal without running the race. Without the race, you miss out on all the memories, the feelings of empowerment, and the sense of victory. At the same time, you don't just wake up one day and say, "Today I am running a marathon!" If you did, the odds are that you wouldn't be able to finish, at least not without injury. Running a marathon is about endurance. People train for up to a year to get ready to run those 26.2 miles. I believe we need to prepare ourselves for pregnancy in the same way.

While helping women throughout their pregnancies, I have found that there is a direct correlation between how much you prepare for your pregnancy, your enjoyment of it, and the success of your birth plan. But unfortunately, most women don't get ready. We must prepare our bodies for this 40-week journey just like an aspiring marathoner trains for months. Doing this will not only increase your chances of fully enjoying your pregnancy, but will also help you get a rock-solid body once your baby is born.

If you are already pregnant, you may be tempted to skip the chapter **Preheating the Oven** where we discuss the basics of preparing for conception because you think it's too late for you. However, I encourage you to read it so that you may apply this knowledge to future pregnancies or help expecting moms in your family, circle of friends, or just about anyone who will allow you to! This is very valuable information and if your first-born is anything like mine, it will be difficult to find quiet moments to read after he or she is born. I read many books during my first pregnancy and none in preparation for my second one. You will find that even going to the rest room is an open event when you have a toddler!

Every pregnancy is unique; resist the temptation to compare your pregnancies. I believe you can have your best possible pregnancy if you are equipped with knowledge and will power. My goal is that you find both in this book. You will also find helpful information on the following:

- true nutrition;
- exercising through all three trimesters and beyond;
- the importance of rest and how it helps accomplish your busy schedule;
- chiropractic and naturopathic care;
- midwives and home births as the best way to achieve a natural birth; and
- bouncing back to your pre-pregnancy weight.

All in an easy-to-read format that allows you to always come back to the book and easily

find what you're looking for. I also mention many of my favorite products in this book. I don't profit from any of these recommendations. I just want you to know what has worked well for me.

You should read this book cover to cover in order to get the most out of it. Every part of it is important in passing on to you the understanding of true health and how it translates into a healthy pregnancy, baby, and birth. Implementing what you learn and becoming **truly healthy** will not only help you enjoy your pregnancy to the fullest, but will also help you be healthy and remain healthy after you deliver.

Thank you for deciding to read my book in preparation for your pregnancy. I wrote it with you in mind at all times. I hope you enjoy every page, every story, and every word.

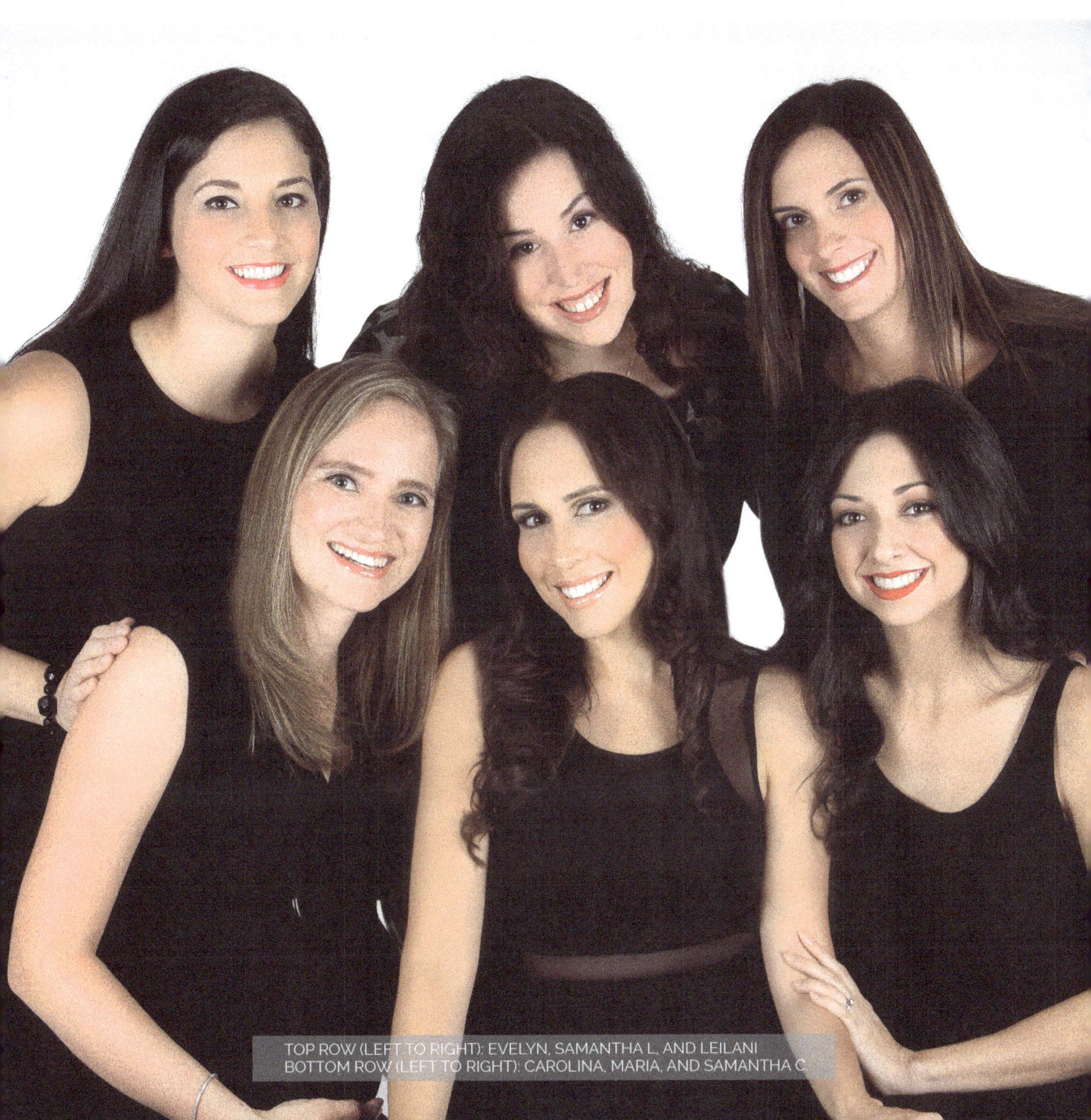

TOP ROW (LEFT TO RIGHT): EVELYN, SAMANTHA L, AND LEILANI
BOTTOM ROW (LEFT TO RIGHT): CAROLINA, MARIA, AND SAMANTHA C.

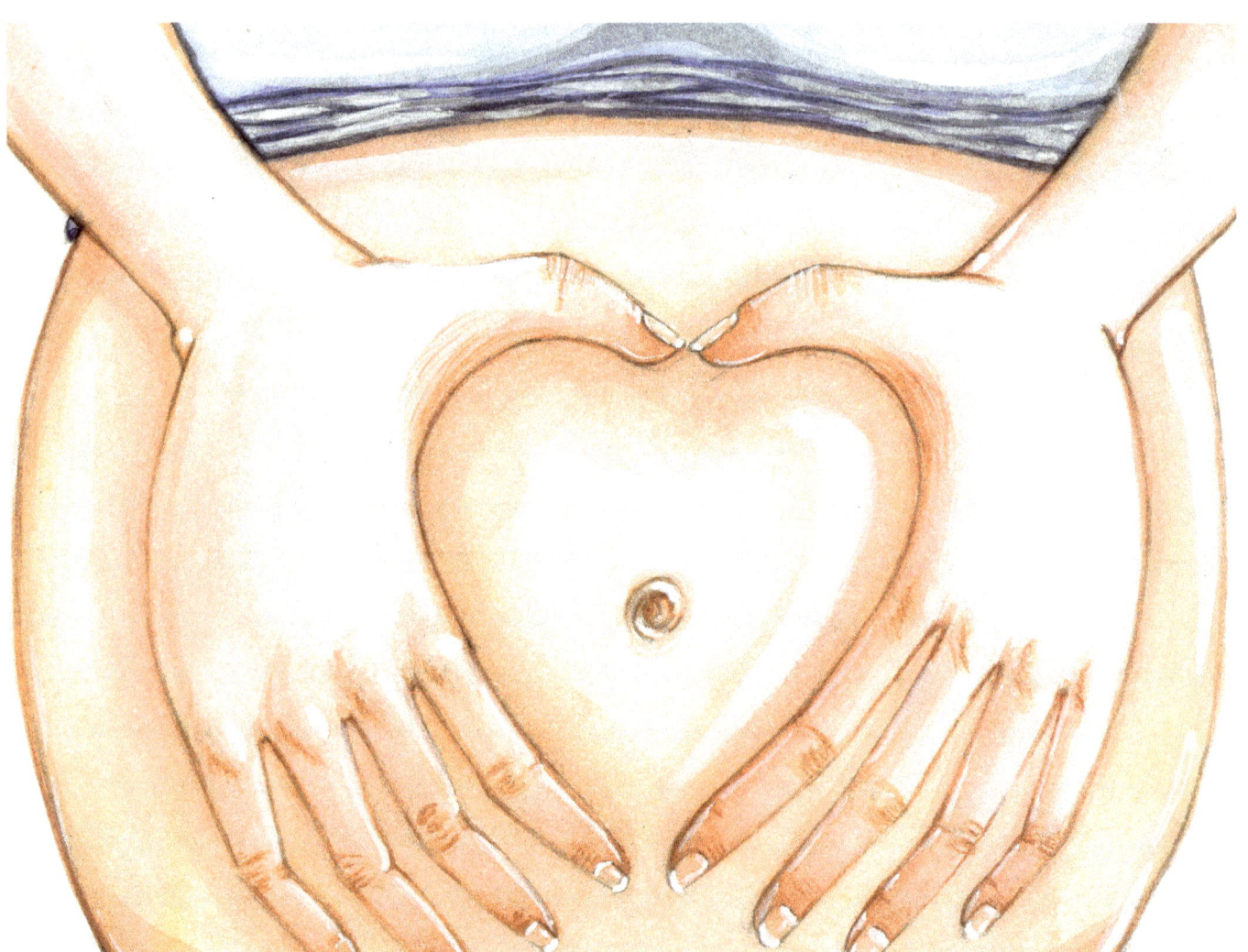

CHAPTER 1
Preheating the Oven

Leilani tried to conceive for almost a year. She was 27 years old at the time and looked perfectly healthy. She was even in great shape—she just couldn't get pregnant. As a registered nurse, Leilani was very knowledgeable about health. When she found out she had polycystic ovary syndrome (PCOS), she sought treatment from her OB/GYN, who told her to go back on birth control as a way to treat the PCOS.

"I had cysts everywhere!" she remembers, "But taking birth control didn't seem right. I wanted to get pregnant. Why would I go back on birth control?" She knew a naturopath and decided to give alternative treatment a chance. She visited Dr. Gisela Hernandez, in Aventura, Florida, and began naturopathic treatment. Thirty days later, she was pregnant. Leilani now has three beautiful children.

Cecilia is another woman who, like Leilani, had struggled to conceive. She tried for seven years. She had undergone various testing with an OB/GYN and a fertility specialist and learned that she did not ovulate consistently. They first prescribed her different hormones that made her aggressive, depressed, and volatile. After that didn't work, she tried artificial insemination, but still to no avail.

Cecilia was also seeing a gastroenterologist due to pain in her gallbladder. She recalls, "According to God's perfect plan, my co-worker told me about Dr. Hernandez. During my preliminary evaluation, Dr. Hernandez examined my iris and found that I had gallstones. She followed up by asking me if I had any children, at which point I started crying. I was in awe that she had pin-

pointed everything my body was struggling with." Dr. Hernandez explained to her that she would not be able to conceive until her gallbladder healed. Cecilia cleansed her body of the excess hormones caused by the fertility treatments, got rid of the gallstones quickly and naturally, and enhanced her reproductive system. She became pregnant with her precious daughter, Cecilia Maria, after just six months of naturopathic treatment.

A naturopath addresses whatever health issues are hindering a woman from conceiving. This is especially helpful for women with preexisting conditions—it is better to address those illnesses during preheating in order to aid in conception and avoid a difficult pregnancy. Leilani and Cecilia's bodies wouldn't allow them to get pregnant until they addressed their underlying health issues.

Sometimes a woman's body needs to detox before pregnancy. Dr. Hernandez says, "The liver or nervous system may need special care before conception is possible." Visiting a naturopath in preparation for pregnancy will help you make sure that your body is ready to begin pregnancy. Naturopaths may use diagnostic techniques, such as iridology—the study of your eye's iris—to determine what organs in your body need to be addressed. They can also recommend a prenatal that is right for you. Naturopaths aren't covered by insurance, but are well worth the investment—especially when addressing fertility and when the alternative is an expensive IVF treatment.

Visiting a chiropractor before conception will begin strengthening all the systems in your body so that you remain strong once you conceive, and subsequently throughout your preg-

Getting checked by a chiropractor is just as important in preparation for conception. My chiropractor, Dr. Joe Coffman, puts it this way,

> *Your spinal cord is like a river, carrying life energy from your brain, through your spine, to all the vital organs and tissues of your body. Each and every organ (including your reproductive organs) is totally dependent on that energy to keep YOU alive and healthy. And as soon as you conceive you'll essentially have another "organ," your baby, and he or she will be totally dependent on that neurological energy to develop, grow, and thrive.*

nancy. You can find a list of recommended chiropractors that have undergone additional training to better serve mothers and children at *www.icpa4kids.com*. Chapter 7 has more information on how to choose a good chiropractor.

Preheating the oven isn't only about helping you conceive. It's also about making sure you are in optimal health for and during pregnancy. Your immune system is weakened when you conceive, and many other conditions like allergies and respiratory problems that were under control could resurface. By preparing your body before conception, you will be strengthening your immune system and become better equipped to manage first trimester symptoms that affect so many women.

Your baby's most critical development takes place during the first three months; your baby is fully formed by the end of those first twelve weeks of pregnancy. However, a lot of women don't even know they are pregnant during much of this time and miss out on making better decisions for their babies, like what to do, eat, and avoid. When you prepare your body before conception you are creating the best possible environment for your baby's development from day one.

It is important to preheat the oven when baking a succulent dish or following a baking recipe. Preheating the oven before inserting the raw contents ensures that the ingredients transform into the masterpiece you envisioned. Similarly, we must "preheat" our bodies for pregnancy.

When JC and I first started talking about conceiving, I initially thought the only item on my to-do-list would be to stop taking birth control pills about six months before our conception goal date so that my body could detox. Although that was a necessary aspect, it was far from inclusive. Thankfully, I quickly learned it entailed so much more.

In this chapter, I will share the essential elements for this process. I have structured it in four main areas: Detoxing your Body, Looking and Feeling Good, What to Eat, and Things to Avoid

Happy preheating!

Detoxing and Maintaining Your Body

Detoxing your body involves eliminating any residue of toxins that might be harmful to your body and future baby.

Birth Control. This may seem intuitive, but it's important to stop taking birth control pills or remove birth control methods that affect your endocrine system (the one that controls your hormones and mood). Eliminate anything that will alter your hormones at least six months before your conception goal. I recommend using back-up methods[2] to prevent pregnancy before completing your detox.

Juicing. I heard about the benefits of juicing from my mother-in-law back in 2004. Back then, I wasn't focused on health like I am now. I didn't get a juicer until 2011 when I was five months pregnant with Bella and asked my family for one as a Mother's Day gift. We chose a Breville Ikon Juicer. I had a blast experimenting with recipes and I would post them online. Friends told me to watch the documentary **Fat, Sick, and Nearly Dead**.[3] I only wish I would have seen it before I was pregnant! The producer, Jack Frost, recommends a juice fast to reboot your body into health. You can choose a 60, 30 or even 10-day reboot. This is a great detox to do six months before your conception goal. (Read Chapter 3 for juicing tips.)

Coffee Enemas. Holistic physicians have been using coffee enemas to treat illnesses like cancer for decades.[4] This treatment helps your body make glutathione, an antioxidant that helps eliminate toxins. I remember thinking it was gross, but I realized (with the help of Dr. Norman Chacon) that having all that junk stuck in my colon was much worse. A weekly colon cleanse with an enema is a good idea. I make a coffee enema that consists of one quart of cooled, brewed coffee. Benefits include reduced inflammation, more energy, and better sleep. It makes me feel clean and ready for a fresh start.

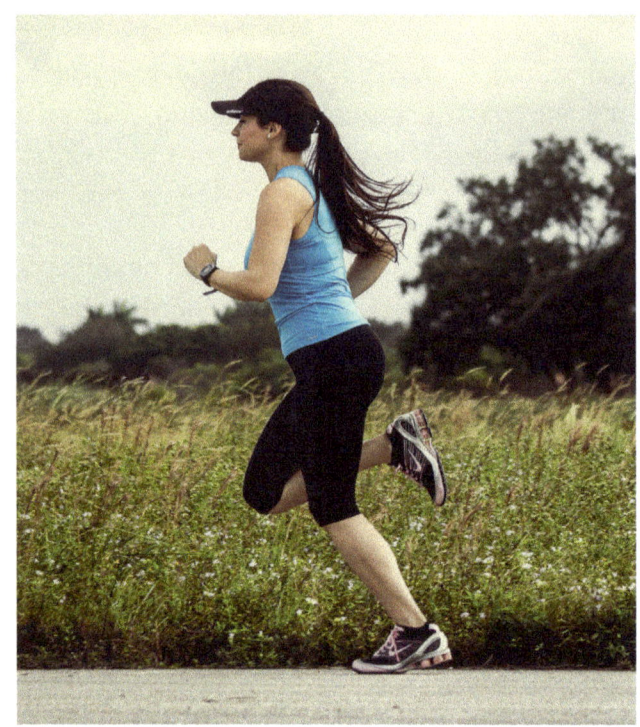

Looking and Feeling Good

This section includes essential habits and routines that will help you look and feel healthier throughout your pregnancy. This includes taking care of your weight, exercising regularly, cleaning and conditioning your teeth and skin, and enhancing your beauty naturally.

Weight Management. A study conducted by Liverpool University that examined the records of almost 30,000 women who gave birth over a four-year period concluded that women who were overweight before they conceived were more likely to have longer pregnancies, artificially induced labors, and require caesarean section births.[5]

Your OB/GYN may not tell you this, but it is so important to ensure that you are at your best possible weight before you conceive. You should achieve this through proper nutrition and exercise and not through diet pills. Find an exercise routine that will be fun for you. Start a workout and nutrition plan that will put you in your healthy weight range before conception.

I got a wake-up call when my mom told me that she gained 35 pounds during her pregnancy with me. I was already 20 pounds overweight at that time. I couldn't imagine putting on 35 more pounds on my 5'3" body. So, it made sense for me to get in shape before conceiving. That way, it would be easier to go back to my optimal weight after putting on the baby weight. I immediately began training for a 5K race with my friend Evelyn. We ran five times a week in the mornings. And doing this together, as friends, helped us keep each other accountable. In August 2011, we ran our first 5K under 35 minutes.

The key to reaching your healthy weight is making sure to establish an exercise routine you enjoy combined with healthy eating habits. Losing weight will be a thing of the past the moment you get pregnant because nutrition becomes vital and so does making sure that you have enough daily calories. So, now is the time to get in shape.

It is important for you to set a goal. First, determine your goal by looking up your healthy weight range. *Babycenter.com* has a helpful weight tracker. Enter your weight and height and you will see your body mass indicator (BMI). Aim for the healthy range, which is a BMI of 18.5 to 24.9. There are different considerations to take into account when defining your goal. How far are you from your healthy weight range? How long should it take you to reach it? Once you have a goal, establish a plan that encompasses both a diet plan and an exercise routine.

Exercise. I recommend exercising at least five days a week for weight loss. You will see how natural it becomes if you incorporate it as part of your lifestyle. You can rest one day after two or three days of continuous exercising with a maximum of two rest days per week. My friend Mark decided to work out every day because taking days off would distract him from his commitment. This is fine too, as long as you are listening to your body and making sure you have a balance. Some days may be more intense than others. You may run or go the gym one day, and do 100 sit-ups at home the next day. The key is staying active. You can learn about Mark's ministry at *run413.com*. Running was very convenient for me, but you should choose whatever workout you enjoy. If you have a pool, you can swim. If you like aerobics, you can do videos at home. Once you establish your exercise routine, commit to it.

Caring for Your Teeth and Gums.
Your changing hormones during pregnancy affect your gums and cause pregnancy gingivitis. It is important that you visit your dentist six months prior to your conception goal date and once again as that date gets closer. Doctors avoid taking X-rays once you are pregnant, so I recommend that you get all your dental work done ahead of time.

Caring For Your Skin To Prevent Stretch Marks.
Begin hydrating your skin with natural oils in order to increase its elasticity. A hydrated and more elastic skin is less prone to getting stretch marks, so the sooner you start the better. Emphasize the areas where stretching is likely to happen, like the breasts, belly, and hips. You will be applying this product to your skin every day, so make sure you choose something you would feel comfortable applying directly on your baby's skin. Skin care products penetrate your skin and enter your blood stream. This is a good reason to stay away from creams with synthetic and toxic ingredients and opt for something natural like almond or coconut oil, which are so healthy that you can even ingest them. As a bonus, they are also very affordable.

Looking the part.
Looking good will help you feel good about yourself during preheating and pregnancy. Make sure you take care of yourself. There are plenty of organic beauty products, such as Miesence. I refrained from visiting salons during the first trimester of my first pregnancy; I opted for home manicures with non-toxic polishes. It is always a good habit to avoid places with strong chemical smells. Safe and healthy beauty products do not have to be expensive. Consider buying items that you can use for multiple tasks. For example, you can use natural oils for multiple treatments and they are both powerful and affordable. Chapter 8 has many examples of products that I love, which you may find helpful. I also share a great tip for saving money and energy when making your purchases.

What to Eat

There is an old saying: You are what you eat! Now more than ever, your nutritional choices are important to keep yourself and your future baby healthy.

Nutrition.
With the exception of being a vegetarian, I had the eating habits of an average person in America before I began planning for pregnancy. I ate fast food meals at least once a day. I had very little dairy, drinking mostly almond milk. And ironically, my vegetable intake was minimal.

The change in my eating habits didn't happen overnight. But I eventually realized that what I ate was vital to my health, and eating whole foods became a lifestyle for me. It was a lot easier to eat healthy once I was pregnant with Bella. My body craved salads and fresh foods. I would imagine Bella eating what I was eating and the thought of her eating fast food meals grossed me out.

Consider fasting from dairy, meat (safe fish is okay), sugar, caffeine, and alcohol for 2 to 4 weeks for a good detox. Make sure that you eat plenty of fruits and vegetables, protein from grains or safe fish, and drink plenty of filtered water throughout the day.

A naturopath can help you design a pre-pregnancy diet plan if you have doubts on whether you can do this on your own. This is an investment in yourself. It is worth it! (Read Chapter 3 for a nutrition guide.)

Nutrients to Consume. **Table 1.1** will guide you to healthy eating choices. The following nutrients are very beneficial to you and your baby during preheating and pregnancy.

TABLE 1.1: THE BEST NUTRIENTS FOR YOU AND YOUR FUTURE BABY

Nutrients	Sources	Benefits
Choline	Egg yolks (from pastured hens), cauliflower, and cabbage.	- Aids in brain development and enhances lifelong memory for you and your baby.
Lecithin	Egg yolks (from pastured hens), grains, wheat germ, safe fish, legumes, and peanuts. Lecithin granules (Solar is a good brand).	- Helps develop the nervous system.
Folate	Eggs (from pastured hens), mushrooms, oranges, orange juice, other citrus fruits and juices, leafy green vegetables, beans, peanuts, legumes, broccoli, asparagus, peas, split peas, lentils, barley, bran, brown rice, cheese, dates, milk, root vegetables, salmon, tuna, wheat germ, wheat and whole-grain products.	- Reduces birth defects.
B12/B Complex Vitamins	Fish, eggs (from pastured hens), milk and milk products, and supplements.	- Develops the brain.
Omega-3s/ Fatty Acids	Fish (low in mercury and high in healthy fats), like anchovy, rainbow trout (farm raised), salmon (wild or farm raised), sardines, and whitefish; sea algae, high quality cod liver oil, walnuts, and flaxseed (e.g., flaxseed oil).	- Develops the brain and immune system.
Iodine	Sea Salt (I use the brand Real Salt).	- Regulates your thyroid gland and metabolism. - It also helps your baby's brain and nervous system develop during pregnancy.

TABLE 1.1 CONT'D...

Nutrients	Sources	Benefits
Natural Vitamin D (Many people have a Vitamin D deficiency.)	Safe fatty fish, such as salmon, trout, and tuna. From the sun and from supplements, such as Nature's Sunshine Calcium with Vitamin D (during pregnancy) and Carlson's Vitamin D drops (for babies).	<ul><li>Vitamin D enhances your immunity to microbial infections.[6]</li><li>It helps with calcium absorption and prevents tooth decay.</li><li>Fights depression.[7]</li></ul>
Natural Vitamin E	Spinach, almonds, peanut butter, broccoli, tomatoes, kiwi, and mango; sunflower, safflower, and peanut oils. If you buy a supplement, know that natural vitamin E begins with "d," as in "d-alpha-tocopherol." The synthetic version begins with "dl."	<ul><li>It's an antioxidant and premature babies are usually low on vitamin E.</li><li>Helps protect the heart.</li><li>Helps prevent Alzheimer's and dementia.</li></ul>
Magnesium	Pumpkin and sunflower seeds, whole grains, some fish, leafy green vegetables. Supplements, such as Ancient Minerals Magnesium Oil.	<ul><li>Helps build and repair your body's tissues.[8]</li><li>Prevents preeclampsia and poor fetal growth.[9]</li><li>Helps against restless legs syndrome during pregnancy.</li></ul>
Alpha Lipoic Acid	Spinach, broccoli, and potatoes.	<ul><li>It's one of the most effective antioxidants.</li><li>Good for brain functioning.</li><li>It also has the ability to regenerate other antioxidants, such as vitamins C, E, and glutathione. So, it helps regenerate these antioxidants when your body has used them up.</li></ul>
Healthy Fats	Olive oil, organic butter, and avocados. Coconut oil is also a healthy saturated fat—one of nature's best sources of medium chain triglycerides (MCTs), which are quickly absorbed by your body to deliver a natural boost of energy (not stored as fat).	<ul><li>Develops the brain.</li></ul>

The Right Prenatal. Prenatal vitamins can help ensure that our bodies have all the nutrients they need to function properly as we prepare for conception. A prenatal becomes even more necessary once you are pregnant because your baby is now competing with you for resources. Being strong and healthy throughout your pregnancy will also help prepare your body for breastfeeding. Here are four things you need to know before you begin taking prenatals.

Take them after your detox period. A prenatal or any supplement for that matter will be counter-productive if your liver is intoxicated. Dr. Hernandez recommends cleansing the liver through a detox diet before beginning to take the prenatal of your choice.

Make the right choice. Not all prenatal vitamins are created equal. Only some vitamin

manufacturers choose to spend money in studies to ensure their base ingredients help the body's absorption of the prenatal vitamin. Moreover, only a few of them choose to spend money on a good vegetable base or animal gelatin. An ultrasound specialist shared that 55% of the pregnant women that she performs ultrasounds on have many undigested prenatal capsules show up on their scans. This is due to synthetic materials used in the manufacturing of many prenatals, especially the ones you may receive for free at your OB/GYN's office.

Don't skip your prenatal. Taking a prenatal isn't just about your baby or your current health. Yes, you want to be a healthy momma, but a prenatal will also help you be a healthy grandma (when that day comes). Pregnancy and breastfeeding take a toll on your body, but especially on your bones, so make sure you take your prenatal. My naturopath told me to take mine with breakfast. I find that taking it in the morning makes taking it easy to remember. And if I forget, I have the whole day to remember and take it.

Check the supplement facts in your prenatal to make sure you are taking enough B9 (a minimum of 400 mcg). I took one capsule of Pro Prenatal Complex ($34/120 capsules) based on my naturopath's recommendation. Take an extra capsule if you are breastfeeding during pregnancy. In addition, I supplemented with 800 mcg of folate to ensure that I absorbed a sufficient amount. The next section explains the importance of folate starting at preheating.

Supplement with Folate instead of Folic Acid. Folate, also known as B9, is the natural form of its popular synthetic version folic acid. Folate is important for mom and baby before conception and during pregnancy, particularly during the first trimester when the baby's brain, spinal cord, heart, and organs are developing. Women who take the recommended daily dose of folate/folic acid starting at least one month before conception and during the first trimester of pregnancy reduce their baby's risk of neural tube defects (serious birth defects of the spinal cord and the brain) by 50 to 70%, and also reduce the risk of cleft lip, cleft palate, and certain types of heart defects.

Folate is also essential for the production, repair, and functioning of DNA. Getting enough of it is particularly important for the rapid cell growth of your developing baby and the placenta, which is critical to your baby's survival in the womb. B9 aids in the production of red blood cells and may also reduce your risk of anemia. Deficiency of this nutrient may also result in preeclampsia, weakness, and irritability during pregnancy.

I took the Folate by Metagenics (About $19.25/60 tablets), which Dr. Hernandez recommended. They are pricey due to their high quality and absorption. I also took a more affordable option, which is the Folate by Solgar ($5.75/100 tablets).

Things to Avoid

When "two roads diverged in a wood... I took the one less traveled by," just like Robert Frost, "and that has made all the difference."[10]

Some of the things in this chapter may seem radical, but I know that your future baby's health is important to you. I will give you the facts. The decision on whether or not to take this route is up to you. At the very least you will be certain that you made an informed decision; you took the time to evaluate your alternatives and didn't settle for the status quo—because it is not your only choice.

The Microwave. Use your stove or oven to cook or reheat meals whenever possible. The heat in microwaves is generated by the rapid movement of molecules and the breaking down of molecular bonds, which causes foods to lose nutritional value. So, when you care about having the best nutrition, microwaving those nutrient-dense foods is throwing money, hard work, vitamins, and nutrients down the drain.

There are mixed reviews about the impact of radiation used in microwaves (ionizing vs. non-ionizing) and their effect on your health. Popular sources, such as CNN, have labeled microwaving safe, as long as you use microwave-safe containers. However, CNN did report that a "small study found that steamed broccoli retained more of its cancer-fighting sulforaphane than microwaved broccoli."[11] According to the Food and Drug Administration's website, "The fact that many scientific questions about exposure to low-levels of microwaves are not yet answered require the FDA to continue the enforcement of radiation protection requirements. Consumers should take certain common sense precautions."[12]

I decided to stop using a microwave completely from one day to the next because I'd rather be on the safe side, especially once I had a baby. If I had known earlier, I would have eliminated it during preheating when nutrition is vital. However, I know how challenging that can be. So, consider reducing your use of the microwave. You may find that doing this will be easier than you thought and will translate into healthier and less processed food choices.

Gluten. Gluten is a protein found in wheat (all kinds, including spelt), barley, rye, and triticale (a rye/wheat hybrid). Gluten interferes with the digestive system's proper functioning and is likely to affect your absorption of nutrients. Ad-

ditionally, it is best to avoid gluten if you want to increase fertility. Gluten sensitivity causes zinc deficiency, which impacts fertility. For women, zinc is important in balancing the reproductive hormones, and a zinc deficiency can lower egg quality. Zinc deficiency can also greatly impact the sperm count in men, as it is needed to make the outer layer and the tail of the sperm. (Read Chapter 3 for more information on gluten.)

Caffeine. I went above and beyond what most people do before conceiving. First, I stopped drinking coffee alltogether—cold turkey. Why? I was a caffeine addict. I drank multiple cups of coffee every day. I had coffee when I was hungry, when I was tired, and when I wanted to treat myself. I remember JC telling me that a co-worker told him that caffeine wasn't good for fertility. That's all I needed to hear to look into it. That was the last day that I drank coffee.

But the effects of coffee extend to your baby's health. Did you know that a baby's breathing and heart rate change when a pregnant woman drinks coffee, even decaf, because of coffee's many chemical compounds? Caffeine can pass through the placenta and the baby doesn't have the ability to detox from the chemical compounds in it. Coffee during pregnancy is tied to smaller, later-born babies, and it may even damage your baby's heart.[13] I became pregnant with Bella right away, after I stopped drinking coffee.

Alcohol. I stopped drinking alcohol during my last months of preheating, when we stopped using secondary birth control measures. Developing babies lack the ability to process alcohol through the liver or other organs. They absorb all of the alcohol and have the same blood alcohol concentration as the mother. I wanted to make sure my baby was as healthy as possible. According to the CDC, as well as the U.S. Surgeon General, "There is no known safe amount of alcohol to drink while pregnant. There is also no safe time during pregnancy to drink and no safe kind of alcohol."[14] According to the American Academy of Pediatrics: "Research evidence is that even drinking small amounts of alcohol while pregnant can lead to miscarriage, stillbirth, prematurity, or sudden infant death syndrome."[15] Most babies negatively affected by alcohol exposure have no physical birth defects, but have subtle behavioral and learning problems.

Soft Drinks. I stopped drinking sodas during the preheating time. Sodas are loaded with high-fructose corn syrup, aspartame, and other risky ingredients. I didn't need the load of sugar, calories, or genetically modified ingredients. Sugar is linked to decreased immunity. Drinking two and a half cans of soda (100 grams or 8 Tbsp. of sugar) can reduce the ability of white blood cells to kill germs by 40%.[16] The immune-suppressing effect of sugar starts within 30 minutes of ingestion and may last for five hours.[17] Diet soft drinks are not less dangerous, as they are sweetened with aspartame, whose safety has been questioned by scientists and health experts (See **Table 1.2**).

Acetaminophen and Other Drugs. I wanted to make sure my body was free from all medications—including acetaminophen. In 2011, Time Magazine reported that Tylenol overdose was the leading cause of liver failure in the United States.[18] I also learned from my chiropractors that the chemicals in many over-the-counter drugs can adversely affect the nervous system, thus affecting the entire body. I also wanted to listen to my body and its symptoms instead of ignoring it. I would get headaches during my detoxing stage. Instead of taking acetaminophen, I responded by drinking plenty of water and resting. That would do the trick. You will be surprised how much your overall health will improve if you stop ignoring the messages that your body is sending you and start acting on them.

Moreover, Dr. Mercola, an alternative medicine proponent and osteopathic physician, explains that, "[D]extromethorphan, the major ingredient in most OTC cough medicines, has been shown to cause birth defects in chicken embryos… Researchers feel that a single dose is capable of causing a birth defect and that, ultimately, it could be the cause for a woman to have a miscarriage."[19]

Secondhand Smoking. Many health experts insist that second hand smoke is worse than first hand smoke. Second hand smoke contains over 4,000 chemicals, 50 of which are carcinogenic (cancer-causing).[20] Researchers have found that exposure to secondhand smoke increases a non-smoking pregnant woman's chances of having a stillborn by 23%, and increases the risk of delivering a baby with birth defects by 13%.[21] This research also suggests that secondhand smoke can be almost as dangerous to a baby as having a mother who smokes, at least when referring to stillbirths and birth defects. Protect yourself from passive smoke before and during pregnancy.

JC and I went on a babymoon to Europe when I was pregnant with Bella. It was very hard to protect myself from secondhand smoking. I think the fact that I didn't look pregnant yet didn't help. However, I was not ashamed to change tables at a restaurant if someone close to us was smoking. I encourage you to do this starting in your preheating stage. Your future baby is worth every single ounce of trouble you may need to go through in order to escape the risk.

Toxic Chemicals. **Table 1.2** covers common toxic chemicals. Many of us are unaware of their damage to our health.

TABLE 1.2: TOXIC CHEMICALS TO AVOID DURING PREHEATING AND BEYOND

Avoid	Reasons	Alternatives
Harsh cleaning products	Certain chemicals in cleaning products have been linked to reduced fertility, birth defects, and increased risk of breast cancer, asthma, and hormone disruption. Avoid ingredients like 2-butoxyethanol (EGBE) and methoxydiglycol (DEGME), which can affect fertility and your baby.	▪ Use products from brands like Seventh Generation and Miessence. We use both at home. ▪ It's easy, fun, and cheap to make non-toxic cleaners from safe and effective ingredients like vinegar and baking soda.
Aluminum	Aluminum has been associated with a variety of health issues, including: seizures, breast cancer, Alzheimer's disease, bone formation disorders, and kidney problems. Aluminum is a common ingredient in deodorants.	▪ Opt for deodorants instead of anti-perspirants. I like Toms of Maine. ▪ Never use aluminum cookware.
Aspartame	Ingesting aspartame may trigger or worsen birth defects, diabetes, brain tumors, multiple sclerosis, Alzheimer's disease, and epilepsy, among others diseases.	▪ NutraSweet, Equal, Spoonful, and Equal-Measure are other names for aspartame. ▪ Opt for honey, agave or stevia.
BPA (Bisphenol-A)	Increased research is linking chemicals like BPA and certain types of phthalates to birth defects, ADHD, and hormone-related health issues, such as increased risk of cancer, infertility, obesity, and diabetes.	▪ BPA is commonly found in can liners, plastic products and is coated on paper receipts. ▪ Look for plastics labeled "BPA-free." ▪ Don't take paper receipts from ATMS, grocery stores etc., unless you need them.
Chlorinated tap water	Has been linked with a slight increase in the incidence of spina bifida, when the the spinal column does not close all of the way. In the U.S. about eight babies are born with Spina Bifida or a similar birth defect of the brain and spine every day.[22]	▪ Use natural water, such as spring water, purified water or artesian well water. ▪ Carry filtered water in a water jug, since tap water contains chlorine.
Fluoride	The International Society for Fluoride Research has reported studies implicating fluoride in the rising rates of Down syndrome, chronic fatigue syndrome and sleep disorders.[23] Fluoride advocates claim that the reductions in tooth decay that has occurred since the 1950s were the result of the widespread introduction of fluoridated water. Nevertheless, tooth decay rates declined in all western countries, regardless of whether the country ever fluoridated its water.	▪ Opt for toothpastes like Earth's Best or Tom's of Maine. I also like Xyli-white. ▪ Carry filtered water in a water jug, since tap water contains fluoride.
Lead & Arsenic	Lead causes permanent brain damage, miscarriages, premature births, hearing loss, lowers IQ, and increases blood pressure. Arsenic interferes with normal hormone functioning and causes skin, bladder, and lung cancer.	▪ Get a good water filter. Check out www.ewg.org/report/ewgs-water-filter-buying-guide ▪ Implement a healthy diet; studies have shown that children with healthy diets absorb less lead from paint in toys.

TABLE 1.2 CONT'D...

Mercury	Mercury causes cell membranes to become leaky and inhibits key enzymes that your body needs to produce energy and remove toxins. Pregnant women have the highest risk, since mercury is known to concentrate in the baby's brain and interfere with its development.	- Skip fish that contain high levels of mercury—especially while pregnant or breastfeeding. Wild salmon and farmed trout are good choices. - Consider replacing silver fillings because they contain mercury. - Skip the flu shot.
MSG (monosodium glutamate)	MSG is an excitotoxin, which means it overexcites your cells, causing brain damage in varying degrees—and potentially even triggering or worsening learning disabilities, Alzheimer's disease, and Parkinson's disease.[24] It is also known as: hydrolyzed protein, hydrolyzed, vegetable protein, sodium caseinate, yeast extract, hydrolyzed oat flour, yeast nutrient, autolyzed yeast, textured vegetable protein, calcium, and yeast food.[25]	- Most commonly found in processed foods, but also in dietary supplements, cosmetics, personal care products, pharmaceuticals, and animal food.[26]
Parabens	Parabens are the most widely used preservatives in personal care products. Research has found that roughly 55% of all breast cancer tumors occur in the upper outside portion of the breast—the section closest to the underarm.[27] It has been found that parabens have a weak ability to mimic estrogen, and that the exposure to those chemicals may have an impact in breast cancer.[28]	- Avoid products with parabens. - Other names for parabens are methylparaben, ethylparaben, propylparaben, butylparaben and isobutylparaben.
PVC	Polyvinyl chloride (PVC), known as the poison plastic, is found in plastic products ranging from toys and cookware to shower curtains. PVC is linked to hormone disruption and reproductive and developmental harm.[29]	- Look for plastic products with the recycle symbols #4 & #5 signifying PVC-free plastics. - Use glass jars or bowls to store food. - Never microwave plastic containers.
Teflon	Teflon releases perfluorooctanoic acid (PFOA) when heated to 450 degrees. PFOA is linked to developmental harm and cancer.[30]	- Keep the stove at or below medium heat when using Teflon or non-stick cookware. - Try to use cast iron or stainless steel cookware whenever possible.
Trans-fatty acids (TFAs)	Can cause extensive damage to a fetus and to the brain of the developing fetus. Research from the University of British Columbia shows that higher levels of TFAs in a pregnant woman's diet are linked to a higher likelihood of premature births and smaller babies.[31]	- TFAs are found in conventional peanut butter, margarine, and virtually every other processed food. Trans-fatty acids are also called "hydrogenated oils" because TFAs are created through the hydrogenation process. - Opt for a natural peanut butter brand that only contains organic peanuts and sea salt as ingredients.
Triclosan	Triclosan is an ingredient found in some soaps and deodorants. It is a hormone disruptor that builds up in our bodies and has been found in blood and breast milk. Studies show that it's actually no more effective at removing germs or preventing illness that plain soap and water.[32]	- Avoid anti-bacterial hand soap with triclosan listed on the label. - Reduce your use of disinfectant products. - Check your deodorant to make sure that is triclosan-free.

The Flu Shot. According to the CDC, the majority of flu vaccines contain thimerosal. Some contain as much as 25 mcg of mercury per dose. This means that it may contain more than 250 times the Environmental Protection Agency's safety limit for mercury. Mercury is a known carcinogen (cancer-causing agent). Vaccines also contain formaldehyde (a known cancer-causing agent); aluminum (a neurotoxin that has been linked to Alzheimer's disease); MSG; monkey, cow, pig, chick, and human fetal cells; viral DNA; and live and killed bacteria and viruses—among many other toxins.[33] Yet, the CDC still recommends that children over six months and pregnant women receive the flu vaccine each year.

I realize this is a controversial topic. I encourage you to do your own research, even outside of the medical community forums. Then, you can weigh your options. When people come to me with regrets about past vaccines I tell them not to worry over what is done. There is nothing we can do to change the past. We can, however, learn about it and let it positively affect our future.

Action Step: Determine your conception goal date and prepare a preheating plan for the six months prior to that date.

My conception date goal is: _____

My accountability person is: _____

I'm going to start doing this:

I'm going to stop doing this:

I'm going to continue doing this:

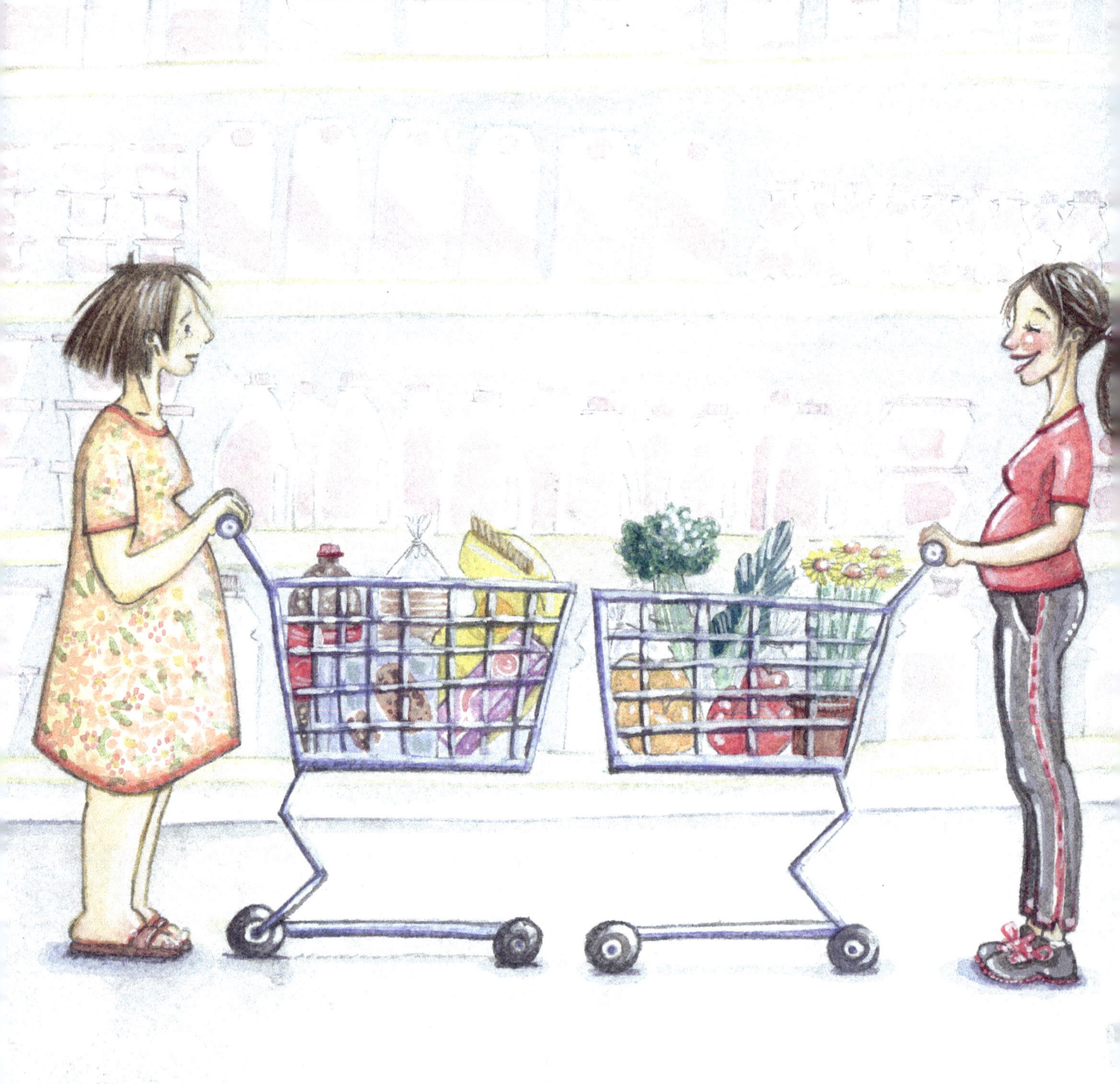

CHAPTER 2

The Hall Pass Myth

One day, while pregnant with Bella, I bumped into another pregnant woman at the supermarket. We smiled at each other and continued shopping. Then, suddenly, I heard her say, "This isn't really good for you." I figured she was talking to me, so I turned around and noticed she was near a table full of cakes and sweets on sale—holding a box of pound cake. I immediately smiled and affirmed her with a nod. I began walking toward her to engage in a casual talk, when she said, "Who cares! I'm pregnant!" She took two boxes of pound cake and threw them in her cart. "How could you think that? You have it all mixed up," I thought as I stood there in shock and still as a rock. I was not shocked because she took two boxes, I mean, after all, they were on sale, buy one get one free! I was shocked at the misconception that she didn't have to care about whether what she ate was good for her or not simply because she was pregnant.

Unfortunately, she is one of the many women who believe that they have a hall pass to eat whatever they want, whenever they want, during pregnancy. Our culture celebrates cravings and encourages moms to wake up in the middle of the night and demand that their husbands run out and buy desserts or fatty foods from strange places far away from home. We get angry with the husbands if they don't do it because "it's their job." We think that it is preposterous to prevent a pregnant woman from satisfying her craving—no matter how crazy it is.

However, we must watch what we eat when we are pregnant more than ever. What we eat has the potential to nourish our developing baby, but can also harm him or her. This is why I began eating so much healthier when I became pregnant with Bella, and my health and body were very grateful for it. I remember getting many compliments about my shape.

I was in better shape now than before pregnancy! It wasn't about how I looked. It was about providing my baby with the best possible nutrition so that he or she could have the best possible start, but I also enjoyed the side effects: I had a lot of energy, was in a great mood, and I looked good.

You (and Your Baby) are What You Eat

You are what you eat—and so is your baby. Your body is your baby's home for 40 weeks. What environment do you want for him or her? I want to encourage you to think about what you eat and imagine your baby eating it throughout the duration of your pregnancy.

I think that will help you determine if you are making the right food choice. Hopefully, this will translate into healthier cravings. Check out **Table 2.1** for a list of creative craving substitutions that I developed to help satisfy those cravings without sacrificing your baby's nourishment.

I never had crazy cravings that I couldn't manage. To be honest, I was hoping I would, but I didn't. They were manageable and being healthy during pregnancy helped me bounce back into shape after I delivered. I was surprised to see that I was able to satisfy a craving for sweets with a plate of fruit. Give this a shot if you want to fool your taste buds so that you and your baby can be healthier! A pregnant woman only needs about 350 extra calories a day, so make them count. I am not saying that I didn't have a treat every once in a while, but I made intentional and healthy choices each day that kept me on track through a healthy pregnancy and prepared my body for delivery. Trust me, your baby will be healthier and you will notice your body changing for the better, even if you haven't eaten healthier before. Your arms and legs may become more toned while your belly grows and your cheeks blush with that beautiful pregnancy glow. You may just find yourself really enjoying your stunning pregnant bod!

TABLE 2.1: CREATIVE CRAVING SUBSTITUTIONS

Craving	Substitution
French Fries	Take organic potatoes* slice them, dry them, place them on parchment paper, and drizzle with coconut oil. Bake them at 350 degrees for 20 minutes or until you achieve the desired crunchiness. Sprinkle sea salt to taste. *Conventional underground vegetables are filled with pesticides. Try organic kale chips. Wash and dry the leaves and place them on parchment paper. Drizzle with coconut oil and bake at 350 degrees for 15 minutes or until you achieve the desired crunchiness. Sprinkle sea salt to taste.
Ice Cream Shake / Chocolate Candy	Try a fruit smoothie sweetened with raw honey. Buy organic cacao and mix it with milk, cream, and ice. Sweeten with raw honey.
Cakes	Bake using organic coconut flour. I used to make a batch of vanilla cupcakes in advance and store them in a Ziploc bag for a quick treat. Toast gluten-free bread, add butter and agave, and then sprinkle with cinnamon.
Pizza	Make gluten free pizza. My favorite one is Against the Grain. Make a quick homemade pizza with a toast, tomato sauce, and plenty of organic or almond cheese.
Chocolate	Make chocolate covered strawberries. Dip organic strawberries into melted chocolate, place them on parchment paper, and refrigerate. You can find healthy chocolate options at Whole Foods or your local health foods store.
Sweets	Your blood sugar may be low. Have a big plate of one kind of fruit (based on mono eating; to aid in digestion and avoid over eating). Try having pineapple, plums, or papaya. You can also have a plate of cereal.
Red Meat	You may be low on iron. Grass-fed beef is a better alternative, but if this is not an alternative for you, because you are vegetarian or don't have access to it, you can try supplementing your diet with a green juice made with: kale, spinach, celery, broccoli, green chard, no fruit, and sweetened with half a beet and its leaves. Have a big plate of one kind of green vegetable (based on mono eating; to aid in digestion and avoid over eating) with a healthy protein, such as fish.
Coffee/Caffeine	Try Natural Touch Kaffree Roma for a delicious coffee alternative. Add milk and honey to herbal teas for a coffee-like experience.

Action Step: Come up with your favorite craving substitution

My most common cravings are: _____

My creative substitution will be: _____

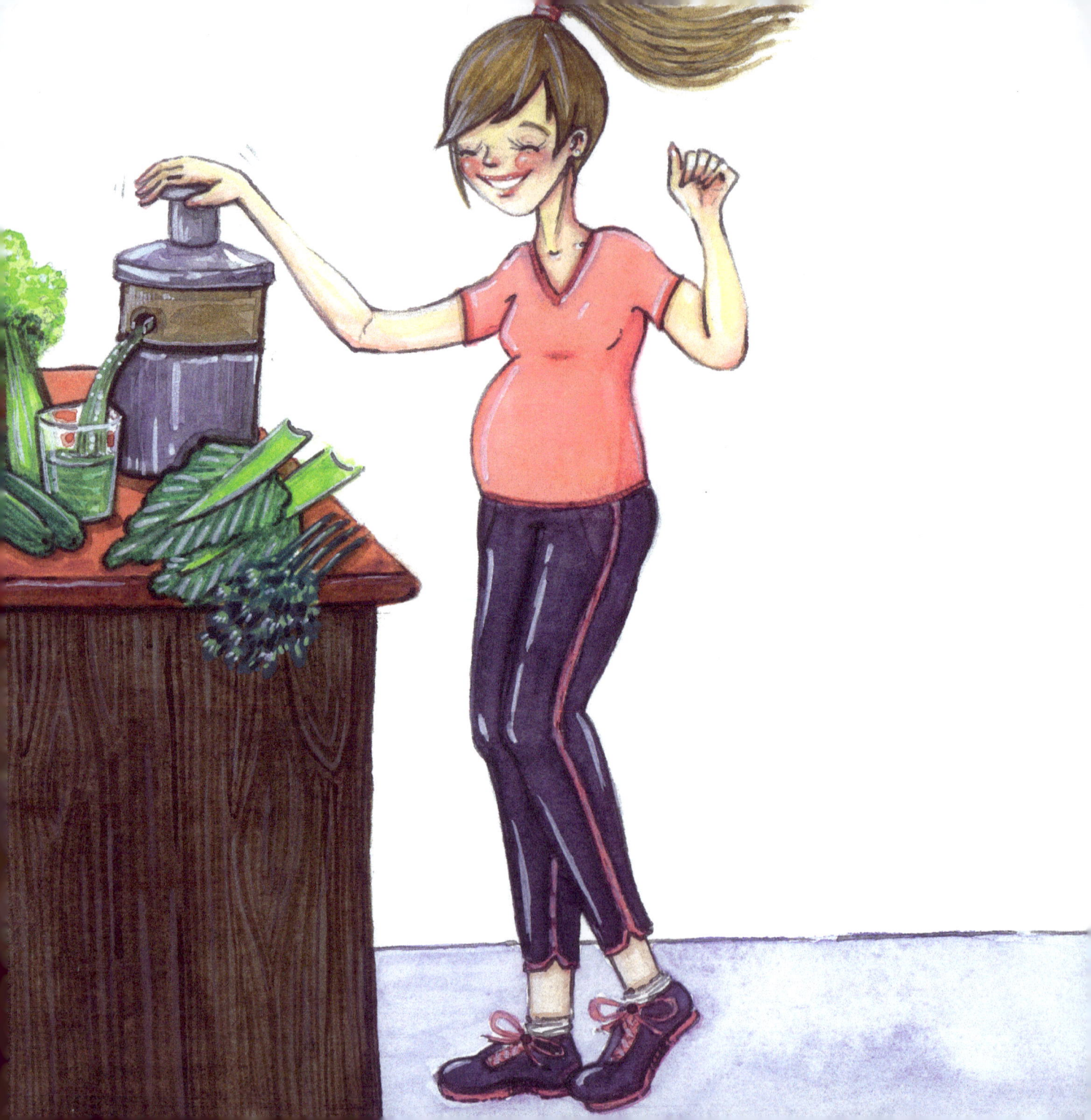

CHAPTER 3

True Nutrition

Nutrition isn't about just making sure that your plate is filled with enough veggies. It's about so much more. It is about making healthy choices daily. Getting into a habit of rejecting the things that are harmful for your body, like sugar, genetically modified foods (GMOs), and unhealthy fats. It's like that saying, "A minute in your lips, and forever on your hips." Think about the long-term effects of what you eat and say YES to your health.

It is always better to eat wholesome foods—the food God made for us to eat. I like how my mom says that the best way to eat is "as close to the tree as possible." This is particularly true with produce, which becomes less nutritious or even harmful when the industry alters it in laboratories or adds chemicals to keep the weeds from killing it.

At the same time, I know it is nearly impossible to eat healthy all the time, especially nowadays when the food industry uses GMOs in much of the processed foods, and very few restaurants use organic produce. Recently, my daughter told me that Krispy Kreme is setting up shop close to our home. I wasn't thrilled. I love those Krispy Kreme donuts when they are fresh and having them (and a blinking red light) close to me is going to be tempting, but I love my health even more. You can have a treat once in a while, but not all the time, not every day.

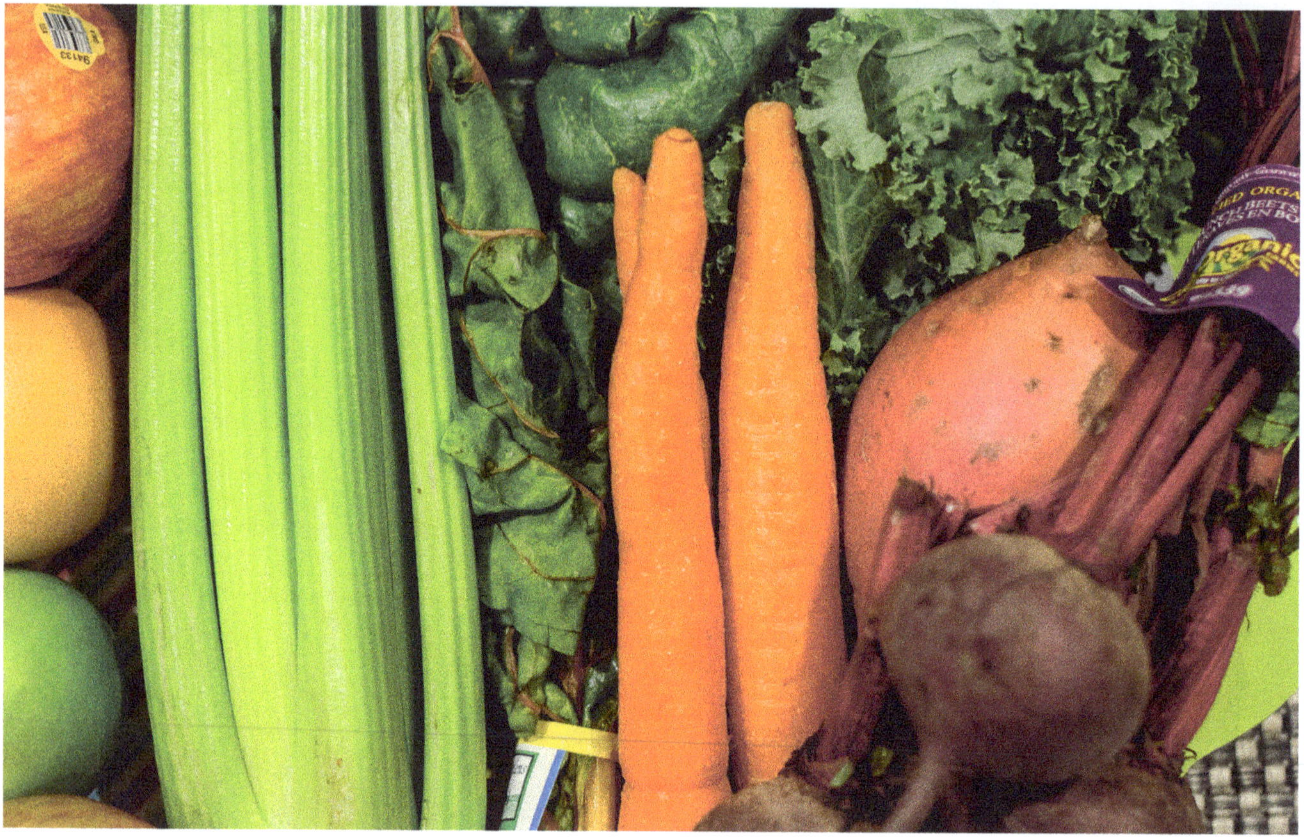

So, if staying away from some foods will make you healthier, how much is your health worth to you? You cannot control what is served everywhere you go, but you can control what is in your refrigerator, where you shop, and what you put in your shopping cart. And that's a good place to start.

I have divided this chapter in three parts: Nutrition and Labor, Your Pregnancy Diet, and How to Buy Organic.

Nutrition and Labor

Have you ever wondered if eating healthier could help you have an easier labor? Most pregnant women are well aware that what they eat will impact their baby's health as well as their own, but few are aware of the implications that their diet could have on the delivering their babies.

I'd like you to meet Leyvis—my hair stylist and friend. She was always in great shape, but when

22 THE SECRETS TO A HEALTHY PREGNANCY

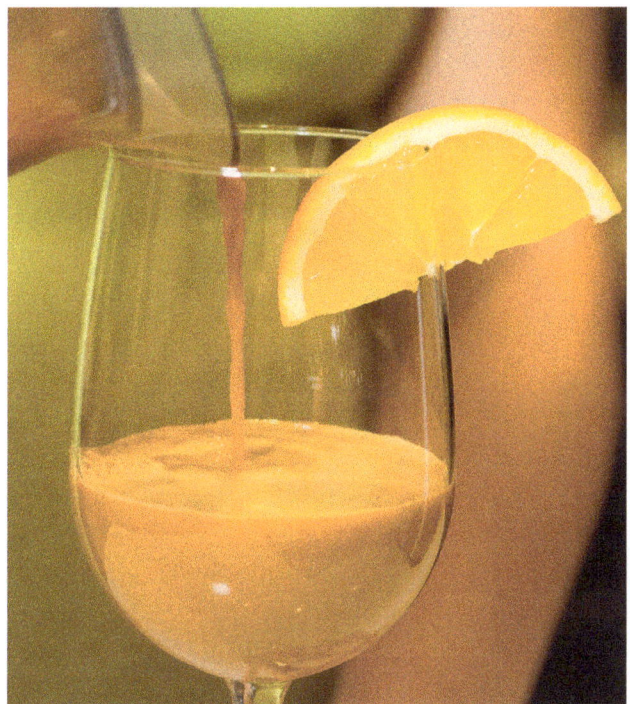

she became pregnant with her firstborn, late night cravings kicked in and she began gaining more weight than she expected. Leyvis wanted a natural birth, so she had sought the care of a midwife and planned birthing at a birthing center. She admitted to me, "My midwife told me during one of my prenatal visits, 'Leyvis, you are gaining too much weight.'"

"It's a domino effect. You start eating badly, so you feel sluggish, which makes you unmotivated to start eating healthy again, which in turn affects the pregnancy overall. I realized much too late in my pregnancy that this is when I needed to be the healthiest. Not just for me but for my child," says Leyvis.

"The day that I began having contractions, I went to the birthing center but, after laboring three days, I was transferred to a nearby hospital. I believe that I would have been able to birth naturally if I had been healthy." Leyvis believes that those extra pounds hindered her from having her much desired natural birth, and in retrospect, she would have eaten better. Her hope is that her story can help women have a healthy pregnancy.

Dr. Sarah Arrowsmith, from the University of Liverpool, conducts research on obesity during pregnancy and says: "Maternal obesity has become one of the most commonly occurring risk factors in obstetric practice including greater risk of prolonged pregnancy."[1]

Nutrition is very important during pregnancy. We must watch what we eat now more than ever. Our nutrition is not just about us anymore; it's about nourishing our growing baby and maintaining good health. Your body is undergoing a lot of work preparing the baby and you for birth. And what you eat can and will have an impact on your labor.

Just like you wouldn't eat a fast food meal before running a marathon or in training for the same, you want to make sure that your body is receiving the nutrients that you and your baby

TRUE NUTRITION

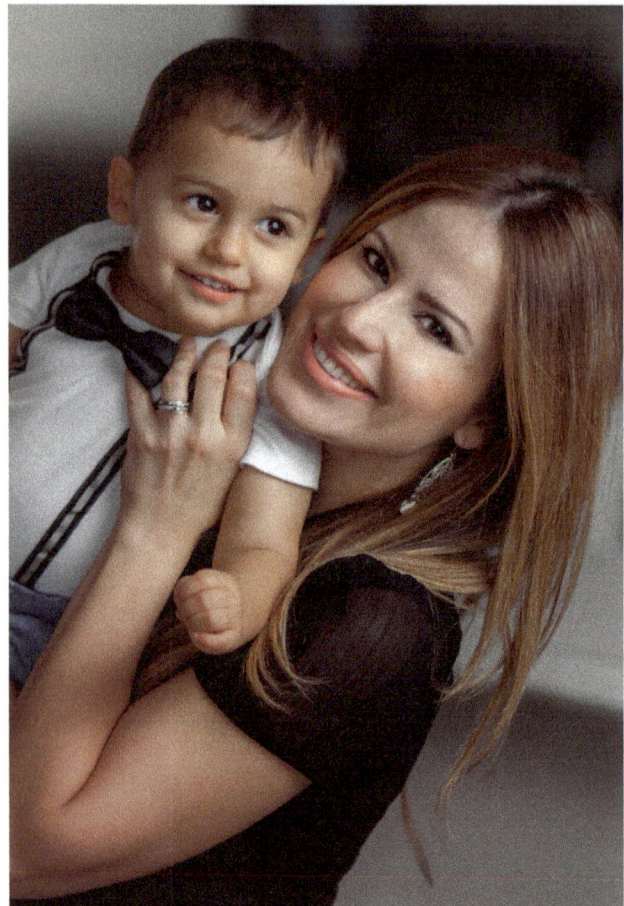

LEYVIS WITH ISAAC, 1 YEAR OLD.

need. The next section provides guidelines for a pregnancy diet that will prepare you for the day of the "race."

Your Pregnancy Diet

Nutrition isn't only about weight management. It is also about supporting a well-functioning body and all of its systems. Your diet affects your immune system, your nervous system, and even your endocrine system. The guidelines in this section consider your needs in preparation for labor, the nourishment of your baby, and yourself.

At around fourteen weeks of pregnancy when your baby's sense of taste is developing, what you eat can affect his or her food preferences later in life. Dr. Miriam Choppard says that a healthy diet during pregnancy is one of the key ways in which you can pass on good health to your baby for life.[2] So, if you want your baby to like healthy foods, start training his or her taste buds from the womb.

Say no to fast food meals. Unfortunately, most fast food meals are filled with harmful ingredients. Instead, I recommend you check out restaurants like Evos, Chipotle, and Elevation Burger (which offers 100% grassfed burgers, gives you the option to wrap your burger in lettuce instead of bread, and even offers veggie burgers). Whole Foods also has a nice selection of healthy cooked foods.

Juicing. Once you are pregnant you should only juice as a supplement to your regular diet. Juicing as a supplement to your regular diet during pregnancy is a great way to ensure that you get many of the necessary nutrients daily in a way that is easily absorbed by your body.

Since the juicer removes the fiber, the nutrients in your juice are rapidly absorbed by your digestive system and go into your blood stream almost immediately. When you juice, you extract live enzymes and phytonutrients from the produce. All those nutrients are easily absorbed into your blood stream at a much higher rate than eating them or blending them.

One or two juices a day can boost your diet with lots of nutrients that you regularly wouldn't consume enough of. Juicing reinforces digestive enzymes and keeps you healthy. I believe that juicing throughout my pregnancies gave me more energy and kept me from getting sick. I would add garlic to my juice as a natural antibiotic whenever I felt like I was fighting a cold. Like flaxseed water, it also fights constipation, which is a common pregnancy symptom.

Juicing made sense for me. It was the ultimate multivitamin that my body could easily digest.

Here are a few tips to maximize your juicing experience:

Use a good juicer. A good juicer will extract the most out of your produce. This is important because otherwise you will spend more money buying a greater quantity of produce in order to get a good serving of juice. In other words, a good juicer will need less produce than an average one to generate a serving of juice. I recommend the Breville Compact Juicer. This Breville model sells for $99 and it is the perfect size.

Drink your juices fresh. Remember that when you juice, you extract live enzymes and phytonutrients. These enzymes and phytonutrients oxidize with oxygen, so it is best to drink the juice right away. If you need to store it, use a glass recipient and fill it all the way to the top to minimize oxidation. Recipients with wider openings, such as mason jars, are also easier to wash.

Use organic produce. Organic produce is free from pesticides. Your body digests juice quickly, so make sure that you aren't ingesting pesticides and GMOs. Use EWG's 2014 Dirty Dozen™ and EWG's 2014 Clean Fifteen™, found later in this chapter, as a produce shopping guide.

Juice mostly vegetables. My naturopath, Dr. Hernandez, taught me that juicing fruits will spike your sugar. So, make a veggie juice—not a fruit punch. I only use a fruit or two for flavoring. You can use organic beets with their leaves to sweeten your juice. The leaves will even out the sugar effect from the beet. I juice up to ½ beet per juice. The following veggies are very good during pregnancy: spinach, celery,

broccoli, alfalfa, green chard (great for iron and B12), beets (for flavor when strictly juicing veggies), and ginger (very beneficial to the digestive system).

Avoid parsley and cilantro during pregnancy and breastfeeding. They can lower blood pressure and don't help with milk production.

Water Matters. One good dietary practice that we often overlook because of its simplicity is consuming sufficient water. Most people barely consume eight glasses of water a day, but staying properly hydrated during pregnancy is fundamental. In order to provide your baby with nutrients, your blood volume increases, and this makes it more difficult for your body to retain fluids thus becoming more prone to dehydration. The effects of dehydration during pregnancy include constipation, headaches, and even more serious ones like premature contractions.

Furthermore, our bodies aren't able to properly flush the many toxins that most of us consume daily (many times unknowingly) without enough water. These toxins are found in meats, dairy, conventional produce, and most manufactured snacks. The toxins that remain un-flushed will go to your blood stream and will eventually reach your baby.

Having a big water jug was very helpful to me during my pregnancy and while breastfeeding. A 64-ounce jug was especially practical during nights when I woke up thirsty and a big glass couldn't hold enough water.

Dr. Hernandez recommends drinking eight ounces of water upon waking and smaller subsequent amounts throughout the day. Although a person's need for water is better determined by considering factors, like weight, height, activity level, diet, and temperature/humidity in the environment, having a formula as a guideline was helpful to me. Dr. Hernandez determines how many ounces you should drink in a day by taking your weight in pounds and dividing it by two. For example, a person that weighs 140 pounds should drink 70 ounces of water, which is the equivalent of eight and a half cups. I also recommend that you continue drinking on demand if at any point in the day you are still thirsty after consuming the recommended amount. A secondary guideline is making sure you are urinating about eight times per day and that the color of the urine is light yellow. Darker urine is usually a sign that you're not drinking enough fluids.

Lastly, since we are talking about water, I want to give you the opportunity to save a person's life through the gift of water. There are still millions of people in the world who die due to a lack of clean drinking water and most of them are under five years old. This breaks my heart. This is why my family and I, together with the support of our friends, raised $5,000 to build a well for a community in Cambodia. $20 saves one life. You can donate at www.charitywater.org. 100% of every dollar you donate will fund clean water projects.

Protein Shakes. Pregnant women need more protein than non-pregnant women. Protein helps develop your baby's brain and develop muscles for your baby and for you (stronger body makes labor easier). Stronger muscles during pregnancy will make it easier for you to bounce back to a fit body as well. Protein provides you with the nutrients and antioxidants you need to keep your immune system healthy.

If you aren't a big meat-eater (like me), organic peanut butter is a great alternative and can also be a great snack with some veggies or fruits. Look for one that only contains organic peanuts and sea salt. Eggs are well known for being the food with the highest amount of protein on the market. I buy my eggs through BM organics and they get them from a farm in Northern Florida called Joash Farms. However, during both of my pregnancies, I turned to protein shakes as a way to get the 71 grams of protein that the American College of Nurse-Midwives recommends as a daily intake. I had a protein shake for breakfast and sometimes a second one as an afternoon snack.

Some protein powders contain herbs that could be harmful during pregnancy like soy lecithin. Look out for artificial ingredients that are harmful to you and your baby when choosing a protein powder. You can use the tables on this book as a guide. I recommend i5 or FitFood Vegan by Xymogen and Whey Cool.

You can also add a tablespoon of coconut oil to your shake. It will harden and become tough to pass through the straw but I noticed a big difference when I added it. I didn't get cravings for greasy foods or sudden rushes of hunger, so I ate healthier when I did add it.

You can also add Amazing Green Super Food. A scoop of this powdered mix contains 10,000 grams of antioxidants. You can have it once a day or up to three times a day if suffering from high blood pressure.

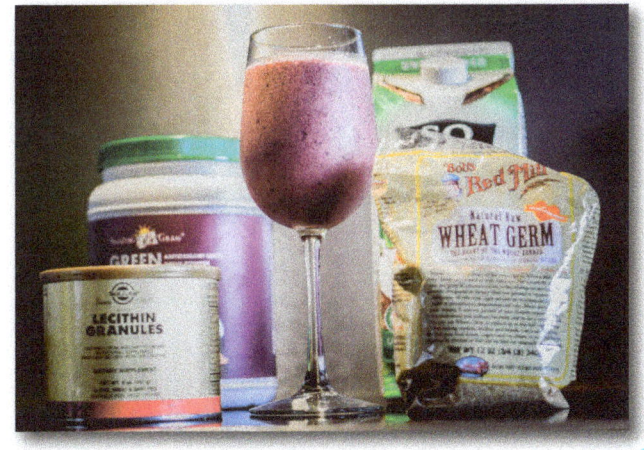

Here are two of my favorite recipes for shakes:

Bella's Protein Shake

    10 oz. coconut milk (alternate with almond milk or rice milk)

    1 scoop of protein powder

    1 teaspoon of propolis

    1 tablespoon of royal jelly

    1 teaspoon of immunoglobins

    Sprinkle cinnamon on top

Mila's Protein Shake

    10 oz. coconut milk

    1 scoop of protein powder

    Berries

    1 tablespoon of lecithin granules

    1 teaspoon of wheat germ

Gluten-Free. As briefly mentioned in Chapter 1, gluten gets in the way of our digestive system's proper functioning. This is a big deal because our digestive system does a lot more than breakdown food so we can dispose of it later. It is responsible for the absorption of nutrients and the fuel we need for energy, growth, and repair. And it is an integral part of our immune system, which affects our entire body, including our nervous system.

Avoid gluten whenever possible. Research conducted by a doctor at the University of Maryland School of Medicine over the last decade revealed that gluten is the only commonly eaten food substance that opens the "tight junctions" between the cells that form the lining of our intestines.[3] Our risk of allergies and illnesses will increase if our intestines aren't able to protect us from foods because approximately 70% of our immune system is gathered around our digestive tract.[4] Our best bet is to avoid gluten if we want to maximize our immune system.

There is a debate on whether or not humans are even capable of digesting gluten.[5] We are certain that at least those diagnosed with Celiac's disease, an immune reaction to eating gluten, cannot. This "undigested gluten" triggers the immune system in persons with Celiac's as soon as it reaches the small intestine—where 90% of the digestion and absorption of nutrients occurs.[6] The immune response can range from undetected inflammation of organs, to allergies or colds that one may brush off as "normal," to painful stomach cramps and diarrhea, lethargy, and depression, among others.[7]

This is why many persons who go on gluten-free diet experience increased energy and feelings of happiness, health, and wellness. A gluten-free diet offers everyone the possibility of a more satisfying life.

It makes sense to avoid gluten during pregnancy because it likely affects your absorption of nutrients. It is important to nourish both yourself and your baby. You and your baby are both gathering resources from the same source during pregnancy. It is very important to make sure that you are able to absorb nourishing foods.

Additionally, a study published in the medical journal *JAMA Psychiatry* found that persons with gluten antibodies in their blood had a risk of autism that was more than four-and-a-half times greater than the risk in the general population. Moreover, every child with autism in the study had elevated antibodies to gluten from birth. It is believed that these antibodies came from the mother's elevated antibodies during pregnancy.[8]

There are lots of healthy gluten-free options available even at regular grocery stores. Check out gluten-free alternatives like brown rice or quinoa pasta instead of regular pasta, basmati rice, brown rice, and organic corn and potatoes. You can also snack on healthier options like cheese, nuts, and fruits.

Below is my original gluten-free coconut flour cupcake recipe.

Ingredients (makes 4 large cupcakes)

½ cup of organic coconut flour (I like Raw Coconut Flour by Coconut Secret)
¼ teaspoon of aluminum free baking soda
¼ teaspoon of sea salt
1 tablespoon of cinnamon
4 organic eggs
⅓ cup of organic coconut oil
½ cup of organic agave or raw honey (sometimes I do ¼ agave and ¼ raw honey)
1 tablespoon of vanilla extract
1 ripe banana (optional)

Method

Preheat your oven to 350°F. Combine all the dry in ingredients and blend well. Add the wet ingredients to the dry ingredients and use a mixer to blend well. Add the ripe banana (if desired) and blend well. Spread organic coconut oil on the cupcake pan before pouring the batter. You can also use cupcake liners. Bake for about 20 minutes, or until a toothpick inserted in the center of a cupcake comes out clean.

How to Buy Organic

There is growing consensus in the scientific community that small doses of pesticides and other chemicals can adversely affect people, especially during vulnerable periods of fetal development and childhood when exposures

can have long lasting effects.[9] Researchers in the U.S. and Canada have found pesticides in the amniotic fluid of pregnant women, in umbilical cords, and in breast milk.[10] So, while it is important to eat fresh fruits and vegetables—due to their many antioxidants that help our bodies eliminate toxins—we must recognize that conventionally grown produce may not be as beneficial after all.

Genetically Modified Foods. Thierry Vrain is a former research scientist for Agriculture Canada. He was designated to address public groups and reassure them that genetically engineered crops and foods were safe. But he retired in 2003 and now promotes awareness of the dangers of genetically modified foods. Thierry advocates that, "There are no long-term feeding studies performed…to demonstrate the claims that engineered corn and [soy] are safe. All we have are scientific studies out of Europe and Russia, showing that rats fed engineered food die prematurely."[11]

Here is **Table 3.3** with common genetically modified foods to avoid.

TABLE 3.3 COMMON GENETICALLY MODIFIED FOODS TO AVOID

Common GMO	Why	Alternative
Corn	Several studies have shown regular dietary consumption of GMO version of corn leads to serious health problems and negatively affects the kidney and liver, as well as the heart, adrenal glands, and spleen.[12]	Avoid products with Bt-corn (maize) in the ingredients. Buy corn labeled organic. Try a homemade popcorn and coconut oil recipe.
Sugar Beets (Sucrose, sugar)	Unless added sugar is specifically identified as "cane," it likely comes from GM sugar beets. At least 90% of the sugar beet crop grown in the U.S. is of GM origin, which means if any food product contains "sugar" or some other sugar derivative like glucose or sucrose, it is more than likely a GMO.[13] In addition to the glyphosate (Roundup®[14]) DNA, the plants are repeatedly coated with toxic chemicals during their growing cycle.[15]	The best way to avoid sugar beets is to avoid products with sucrose (sugar). Always look for "cane sugar," or preferably "evaporated cane juice," in order to avoid GM sugar. Raw agave nectar, pure stevia extract, and xylitol are also safe, non-GMO sugar and sugar substitutes.
Artificial sweeteners, like Aspartame	If it contains artificial sweetener, it likely contains GMOs. According to the United States Environmental Protection Agency, aspartame causes neurotoxicity.[16] This means it poisons or damages nerve tissue[17]	I like organic agave or raw honey.
HFCS (High Fructose Corn Syrup)	HFCS is made from corn, which is likely to be a GMO strain. It then goes through a process involving bacterial enzymes and fungus. It also contains mercury. Princeton and Oxford have linked HFCS to weight gain and Type II diabetes.[18]	Avoid manufactured products with HFCS, such as soda.
Soy (lecithin)	Soy beans are perhaps one of the most prevalent GMO products in fields today. Soy has been associated with a wide range of health problems and GMO soy has been linked to pancreatic problems.[19]	As a rule, avoid soy unless it is organic and fermented (such as in miso). And make sure to avoid anything containing soy lecithin.

TABLE 3.3 CONT'D...

Common GMO	Why	Alternative
Corn Starch	Corn starch is a highly processed corn product made from corn—genetically modified (GM) corn.	Avoid processed foods and opt for wholesome produce.
Dairy Products (e.g. Ice Cream)	A dairy product likely contains GMOs unless it is specifically labeled as being certified organic, or as not containing recombinant bovine growth hormone rBGH, which is sometimes labeled as rBST.[20]	Opt for organic "No rBGH" dairy products.
Non-organic and Synthetic Vitamins	Many vitamins use 'vegetable' products as a base for the vitamin. Many of these 'vegetables' come from corn and soy products; many also contain aspartame and hydrogenated oils.	Look for vitamins that are specifically organic or non-GMO.
Beef	Beef feed may contain GMO alfalfa, corn and soy. When cows eat GMOs, it gets into their system and becomes part of the meat.	If you're going to eat beef, it's best to consume organic, grass-fed beef.
Milk	Bovine Growth Hormone (rGBH) is injected into some cows to increase milk output. These cows are more likely to have mastitis, an utter infection that can lead to blood and pus in the milk. rBGHs have been found in milk distributed for human consumption.	You can buy organic milk or goat milk and avoid bovine growth hormones. Watch out for foods that contain milk products.
Alfalfa	Alfalfa is the backbone of the dairy industry for both organic farmers and industry groups.	Buy organic alfalfa.
Vegetable Oil	Vegetable Oil typically comes from corn, soybean, cotton, or canola oils. All of these crops have been genetically modified to withstand being drenched by the pesticide Roundup. Unless the vegetable oil states it is organic, assume it may contain some degree of GMOs.	When it comes to cooking oils, the best option is to find products specifically designated non-GMO. I use coconut oil and olive oil. Organic butter may be an option to avoid GMOs from margarine.
Canola Oil	Aside from concerns about oil made from a plant that's toxic for human consumption, the rapeseed has been genetically altered. As of 2009, 90% of Canada's rapeseed crop was "herbicide-tolerant."[21]	
Margarine and Shortening	These are another form of vegetable oil and present all the GMO problems that the vegetable oils contain.	
Hawaiian Papaya	This type of genetically modified papaya primarily affects those living on the west coast of the U.S. Its GMO attribute is that it's a virus-resistant plant specific to Hawaii and the areas that import papaya from Hawaii.	Check the label on the produce and avoid those that start with "8" which stands for GMO.
Squash/Zucchini	Many squash varieties have been genetically modified to fight off the diseases that can affect them.	When it comes to squash, buy organic. Many varieties of non-organic zucchini and squash are of GM origin.
Tomato	Genetically modified tomatoes have been found to have less antioxidant activity than their natural counterparts. As is the case with GMOs, the genetic modifications result in overall reduced nutritional value.[22]	Choose organic tomatoes.
Flax	GMO flax has been grown illegally. Flax from Canada, as well as from many areas of the EU, may be infected.[23]	Use organic flax.

Source: This table was created with the help of Dr. Edward F. Group, III, from the Global Healing Center, http://www.globalhealingcenter.com/natural-health/top-20-gmo-foods-and-ingredients-to-avoid/ [24]

Recent research shows a dramatically higher risk of health problems from eating GMOs and that toxic DNA from these plants survives digestion. It's even been found in the blood and umbilical cords of pregnant women.[25] Independent doctors at the Department of Obstetrics and Gynecology at the University of Sherbrooke Hospital Centre in Quebec, Canada conducted a new study. The Canadian team told the scientific journal Reproductive Toxicology: "This is the first study to highlight the presence of pesticides associated with genetically modified foods in maternal, fetal, and non-pregnant women's blood."[26] Pete Riley, the Campaign Director at GM Freeze in the UK said, "This research is a major surprise as it shows that the Bt proteins have survived the human digestive system and passed into the blood supply—something that regulators said could not happen."

Even though this chapter is about your nutrition, it is important to mention that infant formula may contain milk with rGBH and genetically modified soy. Research shows that infant diets including formulas that contain these GMOs contribute to chronic, long-term health conditions.[27]

I encourage extended breastfeeding (more information in Chapter 10), but if you choose formula, a healthier alternative is making your own with Weston Price's recipe for Infant Formula available at *www.westonaprice.org*.

Produce to buy organic. Most of us cannot afford to buy all our produce organic—but that's not necessary either. This section explains what produce is best to make the sacrifice for. The recommendations come from the not-for-profit Environmental Working Group (EWG), based on the results of nearly 43,000 tests for pesticides on produce collected by the U.S. Department of Agriculture and the U.S. Food and Drug Administration.

Here is EWG's 2014 Dirty Dozen™ list, which includes conventional fruits, and vegetables found to contain the most amounts of pesticide residue. The higher on the list, the greater the amount of pesticide the produce contains. A detailed description of the criteria used in developing the rankings as well as a full list of fresh fruits and vegetables that were tested is available at *www.foodnews.org*.

Table 3.4 lists the produce to buy organic.

Leafy greens (like kale and collard greens) and hot peppers do not meet traditional Dirty Dozen™ ranking criteria, but are also frequently contaminated with insecticides that are toxic to the human nervous system.

TABLE 3.4 PRODUCE TO BUY ORGANIC

	Produce Ranking
1	Apples
2	Strawberries
3	Grapes
4	Celery
5	Peaches
6	Spinach
7	Sweet Bell Peppers
8	Imported nectarines
9	Cucumbers
10	Cherry Tomatoes
11	Imported Snap Peas
12	Potatoes

TABLE 3.5 SAFE CONVENTIONAL PRODUCE

	Produce Ranking
1	Avocados
2	Sweet Corn
3	Pineapples
4	Cabbage
5	Frozen Sweet Peas
6	Onions
7	Asparagus
8	Mangoes
9	Papayas
10	Kiwi
11	Eggplant
12	Grapefruit
13	Cantaloupe
14	Cauliflower
15	Sweet Potatoes

Table 3.5 lists EWG's 2014 Clean Fifteen™ list of fruits and vegetables found to contain the least amount of pesticides. As a general rule of thumb, thicker skin produce tends to be less affected by pesticides.

I recommend you evaluate the produce you consume frequently. Remember that eating the most contaminated fruits and vegetables may expose you to about 15 pesticides per day on average, while eating the least contaminated may expose you to less than 2 pesticides per day.[28] Consider going organic on produce you consume frequently in order to avoid ingesting an abundance of pesticides.

Understanding PLU codes. The Price Look-Up (PLU) code is a four or five digit number that is found on the stickers applied to fruits and vegetables. PLU codes used on produce stickers communicate important qualities, such as how they were grown.[29] When shopping for fruits and vegetables, your first choice should be those labeled with a five-digit PLU that begins with a "9," which indicates that it is certified organic. Produce items containing a four-digit PLU are considered "conventional," which means that they are not technically GMO but may still contain pesticides and other toxic residues.[30]

PLU codes starting with an "8" means that it is GMO, so avoid such produce.

However, we cannot entirely depend on PLU codes to reliably distinguish between different forms of produce. If retailers don't expect to price GM corn differently than conventionally grown corn, they can label the former with just four digits and omit the leading "8" that identifies it as a genetically modified product.[31] This means that we can use PLU codes as a guide, but understand we cannot rely on them entirely.

If you think you can't afford it. Everyone knows that organic is always healthier and safer, and it is certainly the best option during pregnancy and breastfeeding. However, it can be difficult to buy organic produce and healthier products on a budget in today's economy. The first step to managing your grocery budget is to choose the products you will buy organic wisely. You now have the EWG lists to help you in making better choices.

You can also grow your own produce and can start with just a few items. This can be lots of fun for you and your family. You can use pots to start if you don't have a yard. There are also self-watering towers you can use to grow veggies that you can purchase for an investment of approximately $500. These systems pay for themselves within a couple of months, depending on how much produce you consume.[32]

Many towns and cities have local fresh markets where you can get good deals on organic produce. Go online to search for the closest location to you or ask around. There is a huge community of people who have decided to eat healthier and have created buying clubs and cooperatives you can join to save money on produce. A buying club is a group of persons that obtain drastically lower prices on quality foods through greater purchasing power. There are different pick up points, and you choose the one closest to you. You can also look into cooperatives, or co-ops, such as Miller's Organic Farm. Like a buying club, a co-op is a group of persons that cooperate to save money. Co-ops are usually bigger stores where you must become a member to shop at discounted prices.

THE SECRETS TO A HEALTHY PREGNANCY

Action Step: Go through your favorite foods and evaluate if they are healthy or not. Determine what produce you will begin to buy organic and what foods (if any) you will consume less.

Foods I will buy organic: _____

_____

Foods I need to eat less of: _____

_____

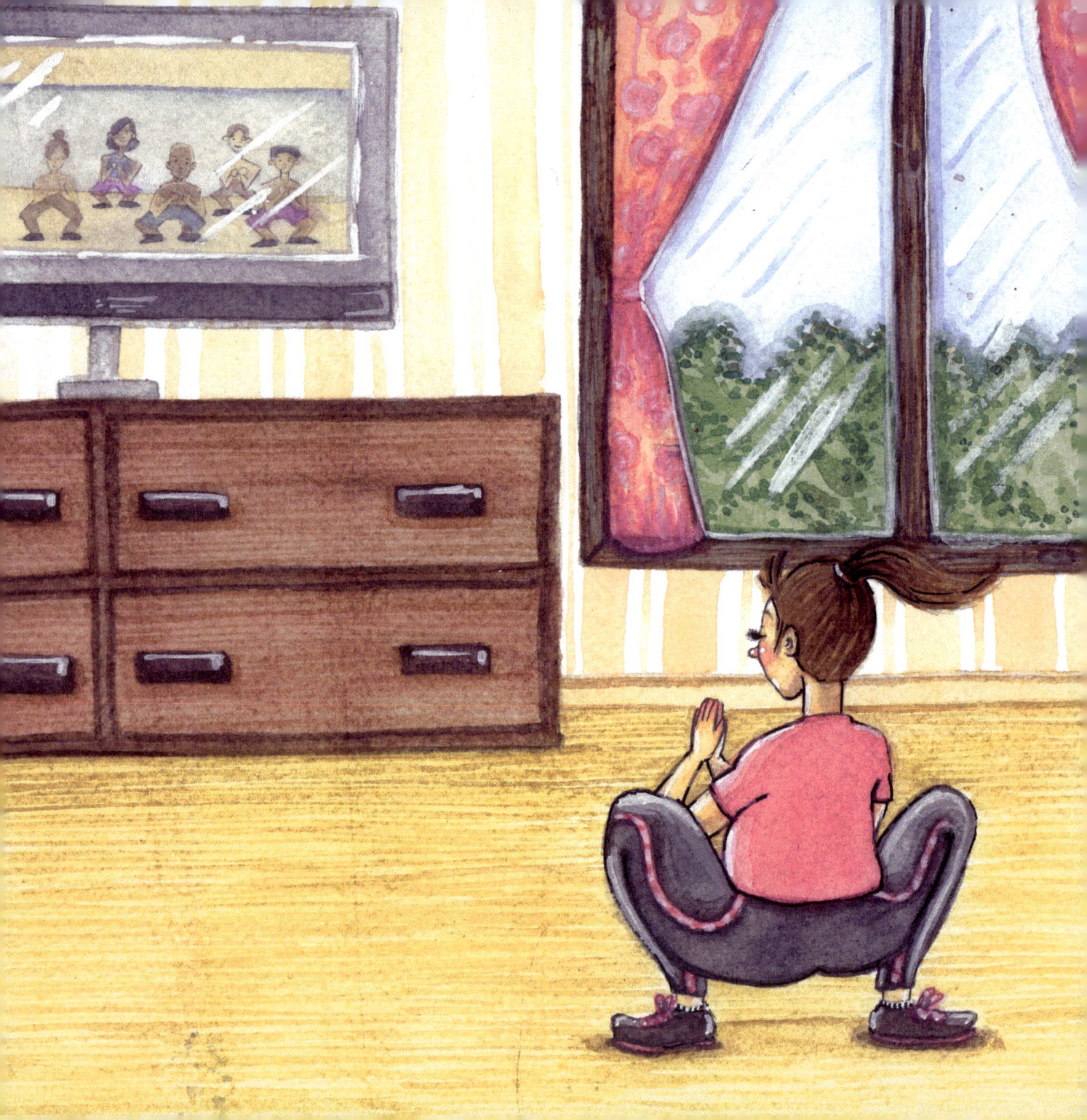

CHAPTER 4

Working Out: From Burpees to Burp-ups

I was 39 weeks and 6 days pregnant with Bella the night before she was born. I remember working out in my bedroom when I realized that I had to modify every single move of the video, and I wasn't really enjoying that, so I turned off the TV and decided to visit my grandmother instead. I had been working out throughout my entire pregnancy, but that night something felt *different*, and I didn't want to force myself to work out. I never had. I enjoyed every time I worked out because I knew that exercise was good for the baby and for my own health and body. To me, working out was an investment in *us*. I always had a blast, whether it was going for a walk or kickboxing with Jillian Michaels.

I received many compliments on how pregnancy looked great on me or how I didn't even look pregnant because of how "in shape" I was, but the best one was hearing from my friend Stephanie that I looked more in shape now that I was pregnant than ever before. *Crazy, right?* But it was true. Even though I was running prior to conceiving, I became more toned once I incorporated healthier foods, especially in my arms and legs.

I also had more energy. I recruited my older daughter Abi and her friends to work out with me and they were surprised at my endurance.

They couldn't believe that even with my pregnancy belly I could last longer than them—who were seventeen at the time. One day, I recruited my mom to do a Jillian Michaels kickboxing video with me. After the video, I went to my bathtub to do straight dips. She looked at me amazed and told me, "You are going to have a quick labor." She was right.

Exercising through Pregnancy is Safe and Very Beneficial

Exercise is safe during pregnancy. According to WebMD, if you were physically active before your pregnancy, you should be able to continue your activity, even if it was running. If you have never exercised regularly before, you can safely begin an exercise program during pregnancy after consulting with your doctor or midwife.

The American College of Obstetrics and Gynecology recommends becoming active and exercising at least 30 minutes on most, if not all, days of the week in order to enjoy the many benefits of exercising. Exercise boosts your self-esteem, helps you cope with stress through the release of endorphins (the happy hormones), sleep better, guards you against gestational diabetes,[1] and reduces other common pregnancy symptoms like fatigue, back pain, and constipation.

Keep in mind that during pregnancy, relaxin (the hormone that relaxes pelvic joints in preparation for childbirth) increases, loosening all ligaments and joints, and making you more susceptible to sprains and injuries. So, check with your doctor or midwife to make sure that your workouts are safe for you and stay very tuned into your body, making sure that you listen to signs that you need to stop or slow down.

I was able to do the workout program Insanity during my second and third trimesters while pregnant with Mila. I would have started sooner, but I didn't know about it yet. Insanity is a workout program that is pretty much like its name—insane. It is very strong and demanding, but I was compelled to join the fun when I saw that everyone in my family was doing it. I really enjoyed how the instructor stretched before and after the workout, which I think is why I never injured myself. I even did Burpees—a squat, push-up and vertical jump combination. I modified the workouts to low impact when necessary and listened to my body. I did squats or hand weights to catch my breath when I needed to take a breather. I did Insanity all the way until my 39th week of pregnancy when my mother-in-law begged me to stop working out because she was out of the country and didn't want me to go into labor just yet. Little did we know that Mila wasn't going to wait for her and my father-in-law, or the midwife for that matter.

THE SECRETS TO A HEALTHY PREGNANCY

The Effects of Exercising Through Pregnancy

Exercising is an investment. Its benefits far outweigh the effort. It makes an extraordinary difference in every stage of your pregnancy and baby's development, your health, and your ability to quickly bounce back.[2]

A Less Painful Childbirth. Exercise during pregnancy reduces stress levels and pain perception during labor.[3] Your body releases endorphins when you exercise.[4] Endorphins interact with the receptors in your brain that reduce your perception of pain and trigger a positive feeling in the body.[5] The American Journal of Obstetrics and Gynecology published a study where thirty-six women in their second or third pregnancies were studied in two groups to determine whether exercise conditioning during pregnancy could elevate endorphin levels. They were monitored and their blood was tested throughout pregnancy and labor for levels of endorphins, cortisol (the stress hormone), and human growth hormone. The study showed that women who exercised during pregnancy had higher levels of endorphins, reduced pain perception, and lower levels of stress during pregnancy *and labor* than those who did not.[6]

Increased endurance for labor and delivery. Exercise improves endurance and stamina, which are both contributors to a great labor. Like I mentioned earlier in this book, labor is like a marathon. Exercise is great training for that long race. Midwives encourage exercise in preparation for natural childbirth because they know that if women are better able to tolerate labor, they are less likely to need medical intervention.[7]

Shortens your labor. A study by the University of Tennessee concluded that women who exercised during pregnancy had significantly shorter first and second stages of labor as compared to those who did not exercise.[8] Labor for first-time moms can last anywhere between 10-12 hours, but both of my childbirths were much less than that. You already know how quick Mila's birth turned out to be and you will read about Bella's amazing birth story in Chapter 11.

Increases chances of a vaginal birth. A study by research expert Dr. James Clapp, III MD that monitored 131 well-conditioned recreational athletes who had an uneventful first half of pregnancy, concluded that exercising during pregnancy (specifically during the latter half) not only resulted in dramatically shorter labors (nearly half the time than those who didn't exercise), but also increased the chance of a vaginal birth.[9] Only 6% of the women had C-sections in the exercise group versus 30% in the group

that stopped exercising. Episiotomies were also lower (6% in the exercising group versus 20%) and active labor was 2 hours longer in the group that didn't exercise (4 hours in the exercising group versus 6 hours in the group that discontinued exercise).

Decreases your chances of an induction. Dr. Clapp also found that labor began about a week earlier in the group that continued exercising.[10] If a woman hasn't gone into labor at 40 weeks, it is likely that her doctor will schedule an induction. An induction increases the chances of a laboring woman ending with a C-section.

Increases your chances of having a healthy baby. Dr. Clapp's clinical study provided evidence that acute fetal stress like meconium, fetal heart pattern, and lower Apgar scores were less frequent in the exercise group (26% vs. 50%). Sweating helps your body eliminate toxins. This translates into a healthier mom and baby.

Helps you recover after you deliver. Lastly, exercising throughout pregnancy helps you maintain a healthy weight, which will speed your postpartum recovery. So, if you want to fit back into your pre-pregnancy jeans sooner rather than later, consider exercising throughout your pregnancy!

Tips to Continue Working out through Pregnancy

Drink enough water. You are more prone to dehydration when you are pregnant, so make sure you drink plenty of water before, during, and after your workout. Stop and drink water whenever you are thirsty. Better yet, drink water proactively so that you don't feel thirsty.

Check out your on demand channel. Check out your On Demand channel for free workouts. Leilani gave me this advice and I put it to great use. I did a ton of On Demand workouts during Bella's pregnancy. Some of them included the duration of the workout in the title. It was easy to choose one that matched the time I had available.

Wear workout clothes. I wore workout clothes while at home and when running errands. That way, working out was very easy when I had the time to do so. I would just turn on the T.V. and go. Cleaning and organizing the house (i.e. nesting) with the right background music was also a great workout for me. And, grocery shopping felt easier with my sweats and sneakers.

Have a Schedule. Have a schedule that allows you to work out at least three times per week. This is not only an investment in your

body, but also in your labor. The more you do it, the stronger you will become and the better your results will be.

Invite others to join you. I liked working out with friends and family. I felt more encouraged around others. It also motivated me to do the exercises right and not give up.

Have Fun! Something to keep in mind as you choose your workout is to do something fun. Working out is not work. Do what you enjoy, whether it is aerobics, walking, or swimming (but no jumping into the pool because it could hurt you and your baby). Make the best out of it. Talk to your baby throughout the workout. I remember working out during both pregnancies and talking to Bella and Mila in my womb. I told them we were getting ready for birth. I often said, "We are going to work out now, so get ready!"

Check out **Table 4.1** for some ideas on an exercise routine. This schedule worked for me. Strengthening your abdominals and core, including your pelvic floor, throughout your pregnancy, will help with your posture and aid in labor, delivery, and recovery.[11] Notice that I did exercises to tone my arms and legs, like squats and straight dips. I didn't want to be big all around, so I made it a point to have leaner extremities.

There is a lot of stretching in the Insanity program. Stretching is very beneficial and I think it helped me have a quicker labor and prevented vaginal tearing.

TABLE 4.1: SAMPLE EXERCISE ROUTINE

Weekly Schedule	First Trimester	Second Trimester	Third Trimester
Day 1 & 5	Cardio/Floor Abs	Pure Cardio Insanity / Standing Abs with Hand Weights / Arms (medium impact)	Pure Cardio Insanity (or walking)/Lots of Arms (lighter weights, more repetitions) and Squats (low impact)
Day 2, 4 & 6	Jog/Walk/Swim		Exercises to open pelvis—lots of Squatting and Stretching
Day 3	Plyometric Circuit Insanity /Cardio with Toning	Plyometric Circuit Insanity / Cardio with Toning	Plyometric Circuit Insanity/ Cardio with Toning/Lots of Squats
Day 7	Cleaning / Organizing / Nesting		

Working Out When You Already Have Children

If you have children and can't take time to work out by yourself (or don't want to), you can incorporate them into the workout. Bella worked out with me when I was pregnant with Mila. She even did straight dips (in her own way) with me and kept count. I also loved using her as a weight during my exercises. You can also go for a walk and take your child in the stroller. I took Bella to the park and we would both break a sweat going up and down the stairs repeatedly. Keep in mind that every minute counts. If you only have 20 minutes, then do a 20-minute workout. If you have to clean the house, clean it like you are working out. The key is to remain active and get the juices flowing.

Action Step: Come up with a workout plan and try to recruit a workout partner.

I will work out these days: _____

My workout partner is: _____

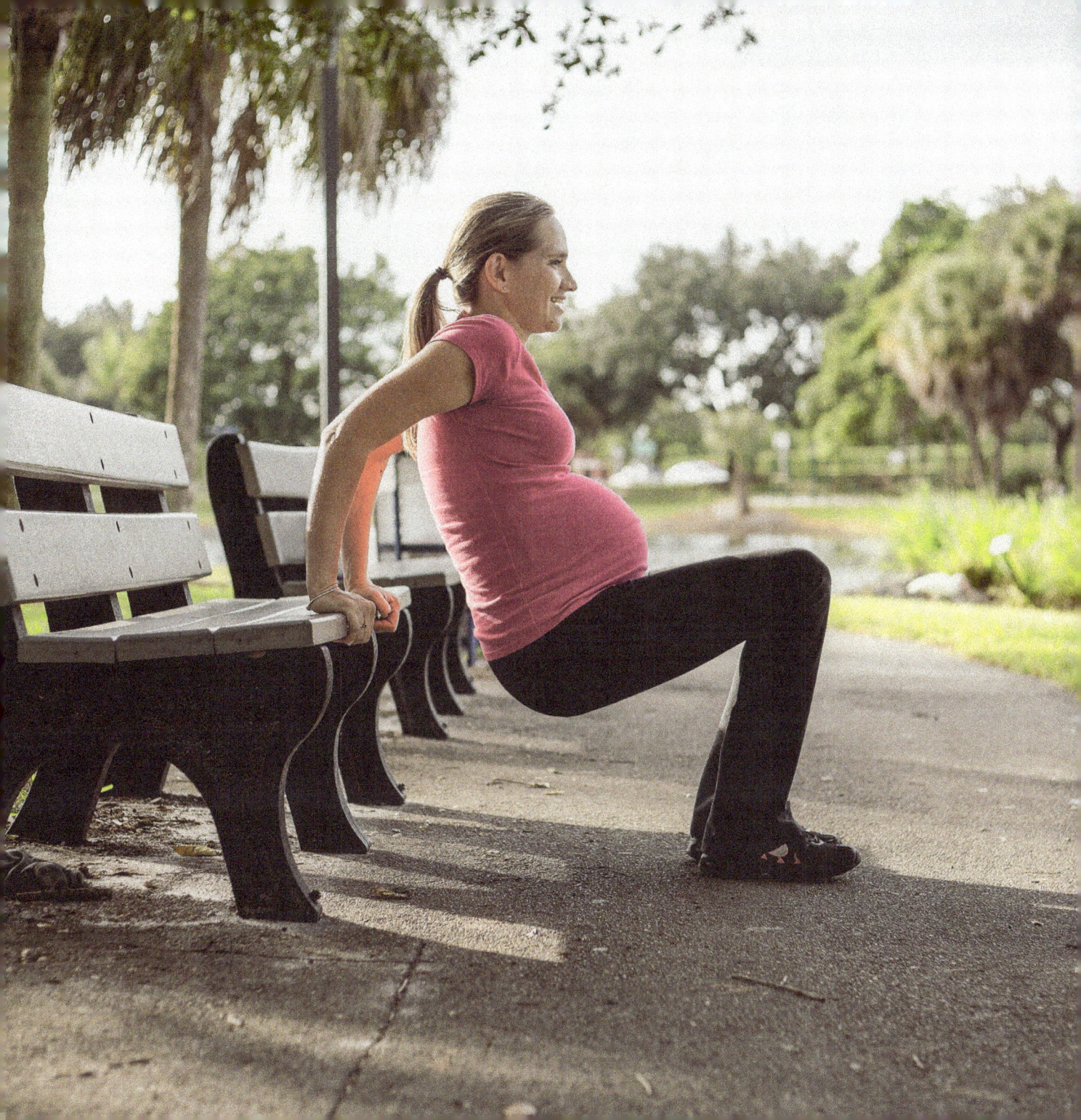

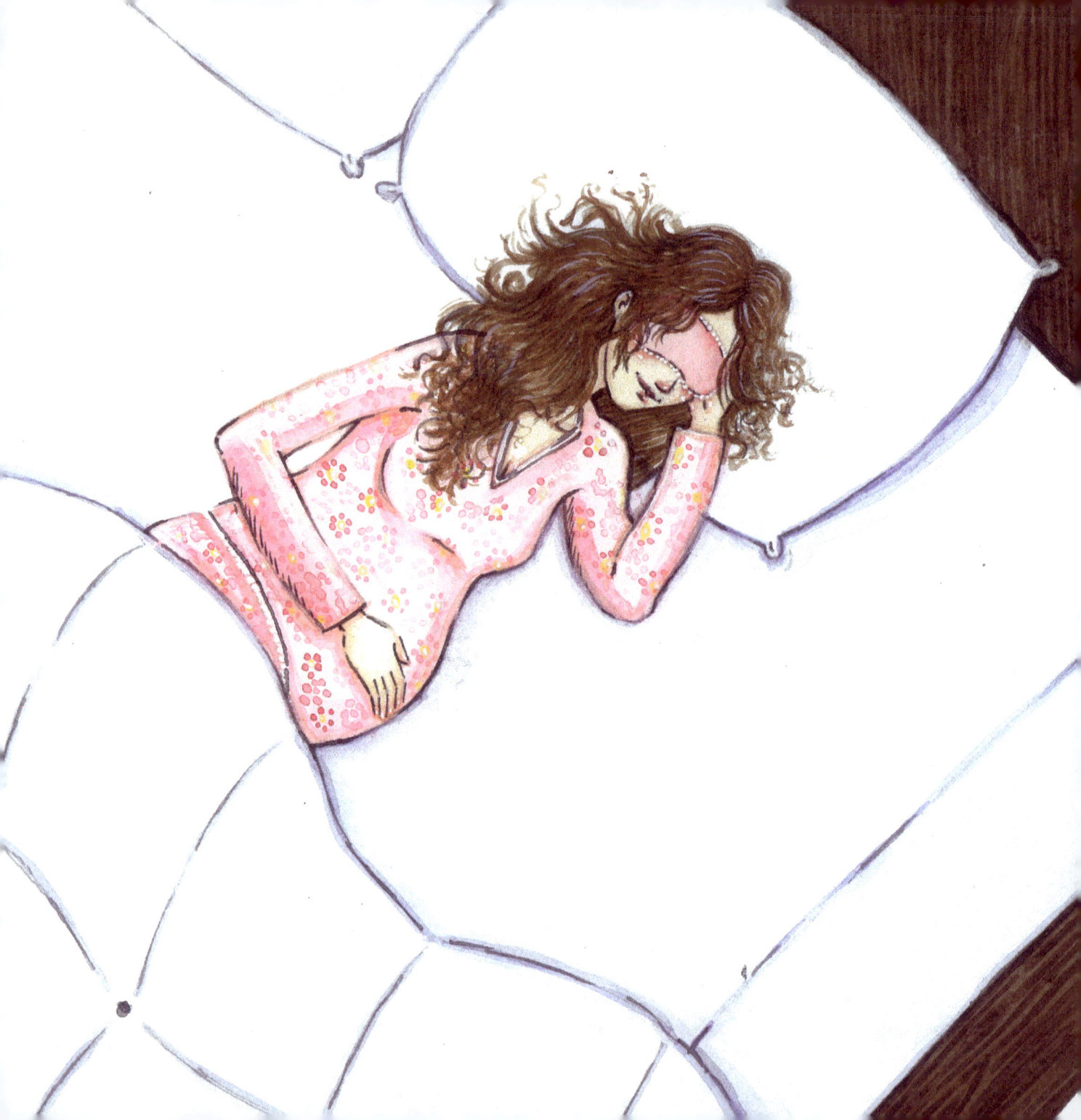

CHAPTER 5

Napping Isn't Just for Babies

"Learn from yesterday, live for today, look to tomorrow, rest this afternoon."
Charles M. Schulz, *Charlie Brown's Little Book of Wisdom*[1]

My first car was my high school graduation gift from my mom. She bought it from one of her closest friends. It was a sacrifice for her and I was very grateful. During my first week with the car, JC and I were going to his house when suddenly my car turned off—in the middle of a hill—in the middle of a lot of traffic—and we were creating a mess. Cars were honking behind us and driving around us. It was stressful and embarrassing.

I was the one driving, but at that point I let JC get on the driver's side so he could figure out what was wrong with the car. I was waiting on the sidewalk when I noticed that JC turned on the car and drove away. I remember yelling, "Wait! Wait!" I couldn't believe that he left me stranded by the side of the road.

I started running after him and caught up. He had just turned the corner into the avenue that led to his house when he rolled down the windows and said, "Come on get in!" I rushed in the car and we made it to his house, which was a couple of miles down the road. Once there, we called my mom's mechanic who made it to the

NAPPING ISN'T JUST FOR BABIES   45

house. He lifted the hood and checked out the car. I remember thinking "I can't believe my new car is already messed up," as he checked the car. The mechanic finished checking the car and came over to where I was. In a friendly voice he asked, "Did you put gas in the car? Your gas tank is empty."

Running Our Bodies on Empty

Everyone knows that it's bad to run a car on low fuel levels, but for some reason we do it anyway. We test how long we can drive with the fuel light on and run the risk of ending up stranded in the middle of the road or messing up our engine. You already know that I have been guilty of that at least once.

We also treat our bodies the same way. We go about our day nonstop until we feel we are running out of energy. Then we trick our bodies with sugar and caffeine so that we can push ourselves a little bit more until we are nothing more than an exhausted body and we crash on our beds and do it all over again the next day.

What we are unaware of is that our days could be brighter. We could feel healthier and be happier—even have more energy—if we just refuel our tank when we feel we need rest. If you think you cannot afford more rest, think again. Just like driving your car on low results in using the dirtiest gasoline in the tank, living your life tired is bringing out the worst possible version of yourself.

An Hour of Sleep Adds Time to Your Waking Life

I began napping five years ago when my husband and I adopted our oldest kids, Abi and John, who were 16 and 14 years old at the time. We were also caring after their three-year-old brother, Guillermo, back then. I was working full time and my routine began at 6:00 AM. I got Guillermo ready for school, dropped him off, and drove far north to my office. I worked there until 2:00 PM and then drove back to pick up Abi and John from school. I then picked up Guillermo from school and began the routine at home. I didn't get any rest until 10:00 PM, when I usually crashed on my bed—exhausted to say the least.

They were worth every ounce of energy, but my lifestyle became a problem when I was struggling to stay awake while driving back from work. I tried munching on snacks while driving and even took green tea pills for energy, but it wasn't enough. One day, I was so tired that I decided to take a nap before picking up Guillermo

from school. I had so much energy when I woke up from that nap. I was able to do everything that I had to do throughout the rest of the day, and I enjoyed my kids more. It made me a better mom because I was happier and more centered. Let's just say that I felt I brought my "A" game that day.

I knew that afternoon napping was what I needed to keep going through the rest of the day. I was in a better mood when JC got home from work, so I was also a better wife. I was able to stay up with JC until midnight just talking or watching TV. Sleeping for an hour added time to my waking life.

Guillermo moved in with his dad a few months later, but we all continued to nap. Abi, John, and I all napped after I picked them up from school. There was no way you could get a hold of any of us at 3:00 PM.

Napping During Pregnancy and Beyond

Napping made all the difference when I was pregnant with Bella. My boss was gracious enough to allow me to break for naptime. I usually took an hour nap after a quick lunch and woke up with lots of energy. I believe that napping was a key component to my high energy levels during pregnancy.

Napping impacts your baby's health.
When you are pregnant, your body undergoes arduous work throughout the entire day pumping up to 50% more blood to support your uterus and growing baby. Your immune system is also compromised in order to protect your baby, so rest becomes critical. A study by the University of Pittsburgh School of Medicine found that poor sleep quality and quantity during pregnancy can disrupt normal immune processes and lead to lower birth weights and other complications.[2] This means that rest is as important to your health as it is to your baby's health.

Napping is a way to prevent fatigue.
Fatigue makes you more susceptible to illnesses, so napping supports your immune system, which makes you less prone to the cold and flu. You are also more prone to stress and anxiety when fatigued, so napping is the kryptonite to stress. It can help you manage both emotional and mental stress. Your mind and emotions are able to collect and many times resolve themselves when your body is able to relax. Naps may just become your secret weapon when your hormones, mood, and immunity are all distressed during pregnancy.

I taught Bella to nap after lunch for at least one hour as she was growing up. I noticed that she got overtired whenever she didn't nap. That also meant that when she didn't nap, I didn't nap either. I got *overtired too* and became the worst version of me, the easily-irritable, cranky, and sleep-deprived Maria. An irritable mom isn't good for anyone in the house. I like to say happy mom = happy home. So, I made it a point to nap for the well-being of my kids and husband.

I made it more of a point to make sure that Bella stuck to her napping schedule when I became pregnant with Mila because I also needed the rest. I noticed that if I didn't put her down for a nap by 1:00 PM, it was really hard to get her to nap later on. So, whenever I had events, I made sure everyone knew that I was going to put Bella to nap at 1:00 PM, whether or not we were at home. I was very strict about it because it made a huge impact on me and my family's energy levels.

By the time Mila was seven months old, she was already on our same napping schedule. Even Abi and John, who are now 21 and 19, still join us for an afternoon nap. JC will occasionally join us for a nap, too, during the weekend. I like to think that a family that naps together stays together.

Naps minimize stress and make you healthier.
Countries that encourage napping, like those in Latin America and Europe, usually score better than North American ones on stress tests.[3] Several studies, including one conducted by the National Institute of Mental Health, have found that short power naps increase concentration and counteract stress that lowers your immune system's ability to fight diseases. This is congruent with studies that show that people who nap are not only more productive at work, but they are also absent less often. So, try adding a nap to your schedule if you want to be healthier.

Napping boosts your brain power.
The length of your nap and the type of sleep you get help determine the brain-boosting benefits. The 20-minute power nap is good for alertness and motor learning skills. Research shows that longer naps help boost memory and enhance creativity. Napping for approximately 30 to 60 minutes is good for decision-making skills, such as memorizing vocabulary or recalling directions. Getting rapid eye movement or REM sleep, usually with 60 to 90 minutes of napping, plays a key role in making new connections in the brain and solving problems that require "out-of-the box" thinking.[4]

Naps have been a secret weapon to many successful persons throughout the years, including billionaires in charge of huge enterprises, and even some of our country's best leaders. **Table 5.1** includes some famous nappers:

TABLE 5.1 FAMOUS NAPPERS

The United States Army	Discovered by repeated tests that even young men toughened by years of Army training can march better and hold up longer if they throw down their packs and rest for ten minutes out of every hour.
President Winston Churchill	He kept a bed in the Houses of Parliament and believed that napping was the key to his success in leading the country through the Battle of Britain.
John D. Rockefeller	He accumulated the greatest fortune the world had ever seen at the time and lived to be 98 years old. He had a habit of taking a half-hour nap in his office every day at noon.
Connie Mack	He was all worn out by the fifth inning whenever he didn't take an afternoon nap before a baseball game. But when he did go to sleep, even if it was for just five minutes, he lasted throughout an entire double-header without feeling tired.
First Lady Eleanor Roosevelt	When asked how she was able to carry such an exhausting schedule during the twelve years that she was in the White House, she said that she often sat on a chair or davenport, closed her eyes, and relaxed for twenty minutes before meeting a crowd or making a speech.
Thomas Edison	He attributed his enormous energy and endurance to his habit of sleeping whenever he wanted to. His assistant said, "[Edison] doesn't sleep very much at all, he just naps a lot."
Henry Ford	He said: "I never stand up when I can sit down; and I never sit down when I can lie down."
President John F. Kennedy (and First Lady Jacqueline Kennedy Onassis)	Head of the household staff, JB West, recalled "during [nap] hours the Kennedy doors were closed. No telephone calls were allowed, no folders sent up, no interruptions from the staff. Nobody went upstairs, for any reason."
Napoleon Bonaparte	Napoleon was a whirlwind of energy during campaigns, galloping from place to place, poring over maps, and pondering strategy. He went for days without changing clothes or lying down for a full night's sleep, but he did nap whenever he had a chance.

So the next time you feel guilty about taking a nap, don't. If these brilliant people napped, it may just be worth your time.

Rest increases performance. For centuries, studies have shown taking a 30-60 minute long nap during the day makes you more alert and focused, sharpens your memory, and generally reduces feelings of fatigue. In the book Principles of Scientific Management (1911), Frederick Winslow Taylor proved that a physical worker could do more work if he takes more time out for rest. Laboring men were loading approximately 12 ½ tons of pig-iron per man on freight cars each day and they were exhausted at noon. After studying the conditions, Taylor

realized that these men should be loading 47 tons of pig-iron per day, not 12 ½! He selected a subject who was required to work by the stopwatch. The man who stood over the subject with a watch told him when to work and when to rest. The subject carried 47 tons of pig-iron each day while the other men carried only 12 ½ tons per man. He practically never failed to work at this pace during the three years. The subject worked approximately 26 minutes out of the hour and rested 34 minutes. He rested more than he worked—yet he did almost four times as much work as the others!

Resting (napping) can make your labor shorter. A study published in Wiley periodicals concluded that nap duration and 24-hour sleep duration were inversely associated with labor duration in women with vaginal delivery. This means that the more the women rested during pregnancy, the shorter their births were. The results of the study suggest that it is important to consider both daytime naps and nighttime sleep when understanding the effects of sleep on labor.[5]

Many women experience difficulty sleeping at night during pregnancy, so napping during lunchtime or right before dinner may be what helps you experience a shorter labor. This is especially impactful when striving for a natural birth.

When to nap. Napping is natural. In one study, researchers had volunteers spend time in an underground room with no clocks or clues as to day or night and told them to sleep whenever they wanted, and the subjects slept in two cycles: a longer session at night and a shorter period—a nap—during the day.[6] It is great if you have enough time to sneak in a nap during your lunch break. I find that napping before lunch is ideal, although many people nap afterwards. Eating fuels me with energy, so having lunch before my nap makes it harder for me to fall asleep. If you don't have enough time to nap around mid-day, consider napping right when you arrive home from work. You will appreciate this if you are nocturnal. Those 30-60 minutes of rest before dinnertime will fuel you with energy. This translates into a more productive evening.

Napping may even help you sleep better at night. According to Harvard Health, research suggests we should plan on adding daytime sleep to our schedule as a way to make up for the normal, age-related decay in the quality of our nighttime sleep.[7] However, make sure that your naptime isn't too close to your bedtime. Napping will give you energy and napping too close to your bedtime may affect your ability to fall asleep later.

Sleeping Positions. "Sleeping on your back is the best way to sleep when it comes to your spine," says chiropractor Dr. Joe Coffman. During your second trimester, sleeping on your back may be uncomfortable and is not recommend after your 4th month. Sleeping on your side (some studies reveal the left side is better), supported by pillows may be most comfortable from this point forward. As your belly grows, the number of pillows you use may increase. I used one pillow for my neck/head, a second one under my belly, a third (long) one between my legs, and a fourth one behind me, supporting my back.

Keep in mind that the pillows are meant to support your body so that your neck and spine are in a neutral position. When your neck is properly supported and your back aligned you will feel refreshed after a nap or good night sleep. Sleeping comfortably will not only help you stay pain free during pregnancy, but also healthy.

Wear an eye mask. Using an eye mask is great for falling asleep quickly whether at naptime or bedtime. I've experimented on the time it takes me to fall asleep with and without the eye mask. The eye mask not only helps me fall asleep faster, which is very important when wanting to rest with limited time, but also helps me wake up more refreshed after napping. My favorite ones are made of cotton fabric because they are warm, soft, and feel more comfortable than ones made of cooler and silkier fabrics.

Take the Challenge. You have the option to either continue letting your car run on empty or give naps a chance. Just know that every time you let your car run out of fuel, you increase the chance of damaging the engine. Continuing this lifestyle may end up affecting your health. You have nothing to lose and everything to gain. I invite you to experience the benefits of napping if you want to enjoy the rest of your life to the fullest.

One hour of sleep transforms me into a happier mom and wife. For me, that better version of myself is full of energy to last up to late hours of the night to spend time with my husband once he arrives from work and catch up on housework or tasks once the kids are sleeping. I find that taking a nap is key in terms of my personal productivity. You have heard about how great my pregnancies have been. You have yet to hear about how much stress I went through both of them. Please know that napping played a big role in keeping me healthy, and it can do the same for you!

Action Step: Determine when you can fit a nap into your day and make a commitment to napping—because it's good for you, your baby, and childbirth!

The best time to nap is: _____

How will I make it happen: _____

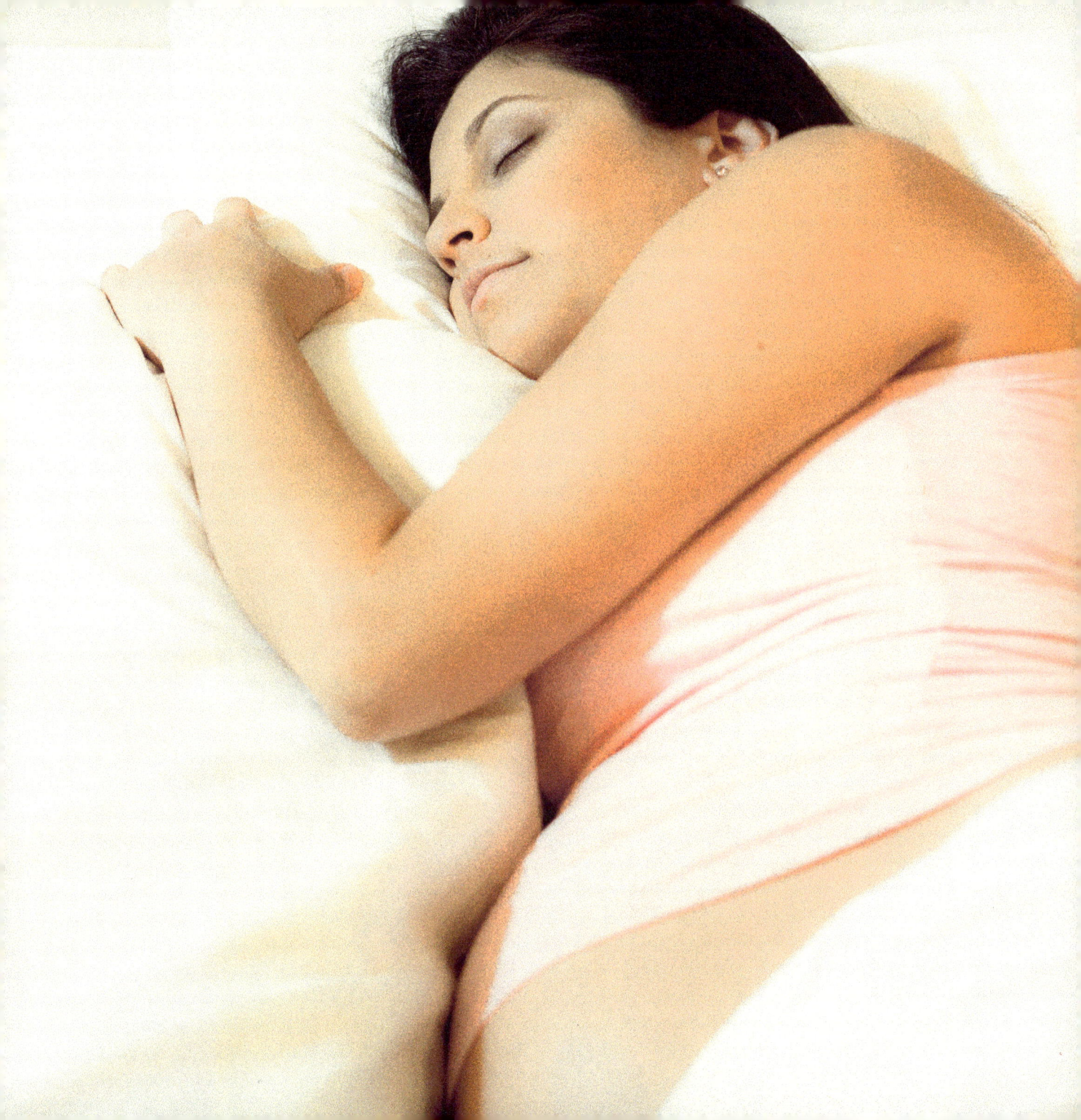

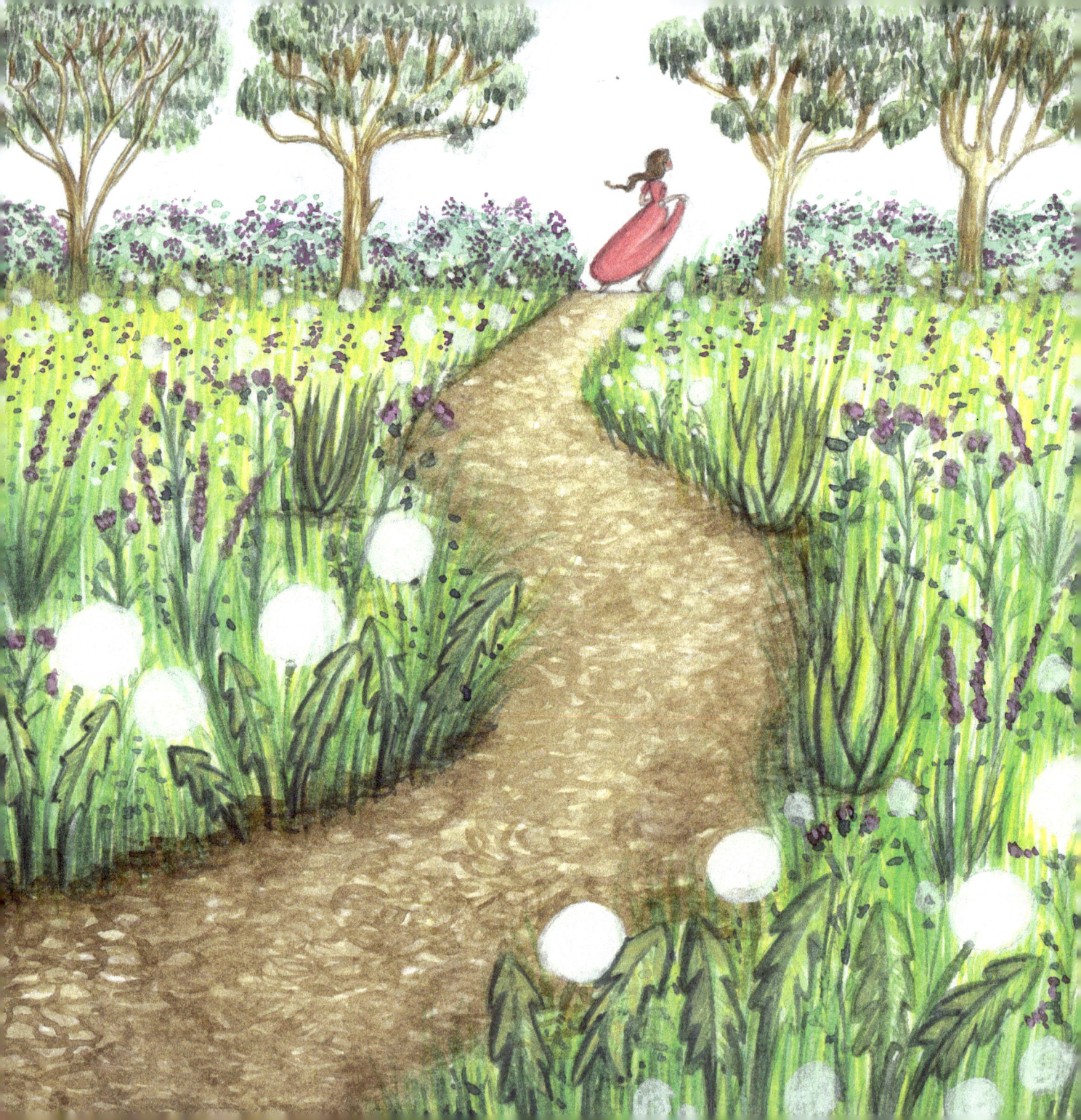

CHAPTER 6

Naturopathic Treatment: The Natural Path

Everything changed one Sunday morning in my native Puerto Rico. I was fifteen years old when I had an asthma attack while my mom and I were at church. Having left my inhaler at home, I was not able to give myself a dose. I was very dependent on my asthma meds back then. I took my inhaler everywhere. I never had the guts to be without it. Whenever we went out of town, we would even take this big nebulizing machine with us, which helped me avoid a hospital trip if I needed additional treatments aside from my inhaler. We were always prepared, except for that day. That day we were empty handed.

As my mom and I headed home, she realized that I couldn't wait for the medication any longer. She was driving as fast as she could, but we were far from home, and it was harder for me to breathe with every minute that passed. As a result, we stopped at the closest pharmacy. She rushed out of the car and ran inside to get an inhaler. I waited in the car, so I don't know what exactly happened in there. It seemed like my mom ran back to the car waiving an inhaler in the air after just a few seconds. She then got into the car and helped me take in the dose of the inhaler.

She told me that she had to go back into the pharmacy after she saw that I was stable. I asked her why and she explained, "Well, I had to steal the inhaler." I made a puzzled face and

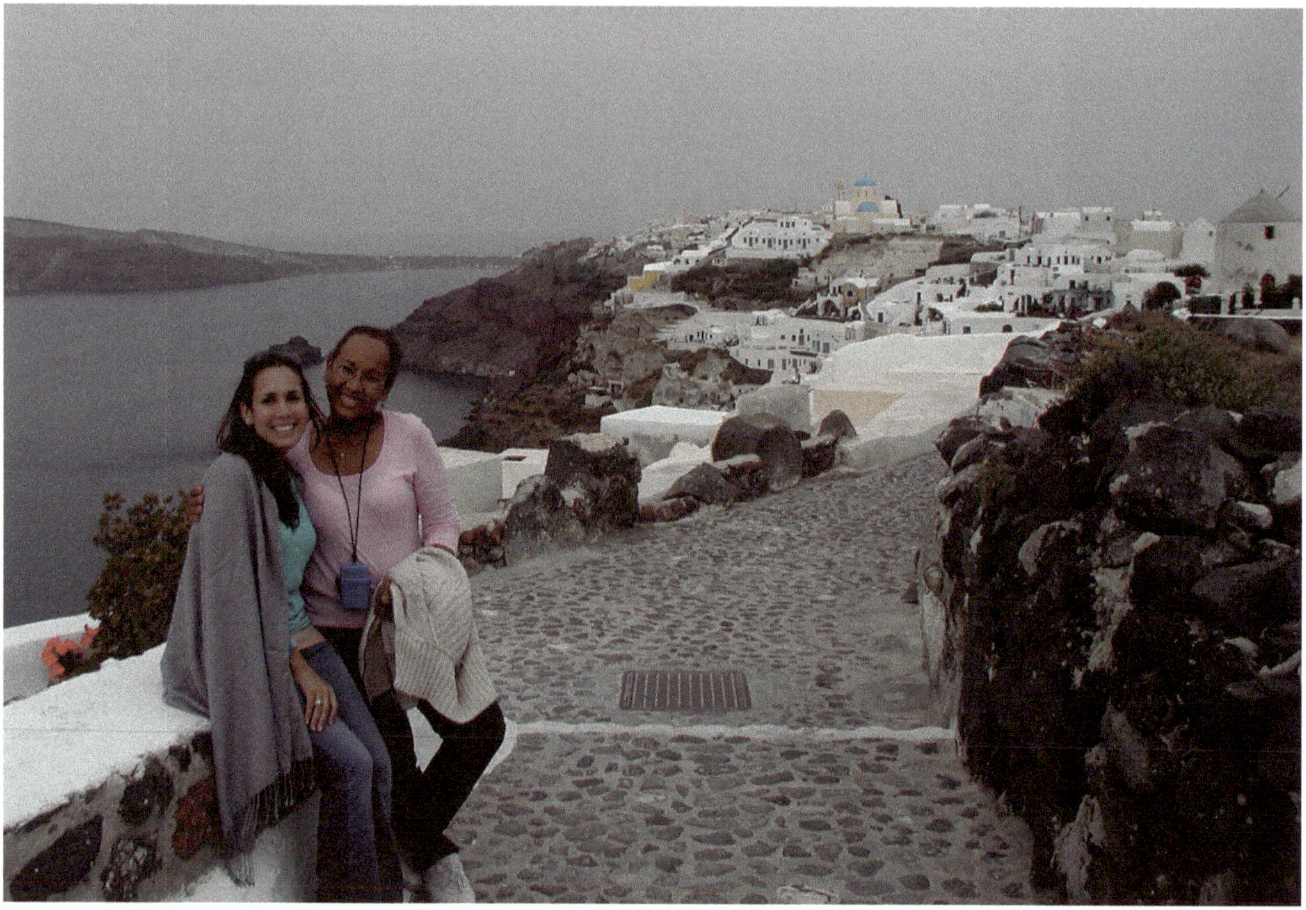

ASTHMA-FREE WITH MY MOM IN SANTORINI, GREECE

asked her why. We had insurance—why would she steal it? Plus, my mother is the most law-abiding citizen I know, even to this day. She then explained that the pharmacist wouldn't give her the inhaler because she couldn't find an active prescription on file, so she left $20 on the counter and ran off with it. My mom was desperate because her daughter couldn't breathe, and she did what she had to do. I can understand her so much more than I did back then now that I'm a mom.

We waited in the car, wondering if the pharmacist would come after her. But she didn't. My mom went back inside, and the pharmacist accused her of stealing. Eventually the whole situation cleared up, but most importantly, so did our minds. My mom wanted a better life for me. She wanted me to be healthy. That day was the beginning of my journey to true health. That day, we realized that we had to try a different route than the one conventional medicine could offer. We needed to take a route that would liberate me from my dependency on symptomatic treatment and actually make me better. We were both eager to try something different.

What is Naturopathic Care?

Naturopathic medicine is about the prevention and treatment of illnesses through the use of methods that encourage our inherent self-healing process.[1] It is ordered and intelligent. Naturopaths look at factors such as organ function, toxins, allergens, infections, stressors, lifestyle, diet, and nutritional status to design targeted treatments.[2]

Naturopathic physicians act to identify and remove obstacles to reach healing and recovery and to facilitate and augment this inherent self-healing process. The goal is to achieve optimal health.

Naturopathic doctors use the least possible force necessary to diagnose and treat illnesses. Their methods include: diagnostic testing, nutritional medicine, botanical medicine, homeopathy, acupuncture, iridology, and muscle testing, among others.

I recommend you visit a naturopath in preparation for pregnancy and at each trimester. You can find a list of naturopaths near you online at *www.naturopathic.org*.

Naturopathic care as a cure to illness.

My first Naturopath was Dr. Norman Gonzalez Chacon in San Juan, PR. He completely eliminated my dependency on my inhaler. I didn't have a need for the inhaler once I started naturopathic treatment with him. He told me to use it if I needed it, but I didn't need it anymore. He made a huge impact on my health then and thereafter. I still remember the things he taught me in the very beginning of my treatment. He was so good at educating me and encouraging me throughout my healing process. I understood naturopathic care and embraced it at only 15 years old.

Dr. Norman used iridology to diagnose and monitor the success of his treatment. Iridology is the study of the iris of the eye—the exposed nerve endings that make up the colored part of the eye. The iris is like a map of the body. Specific parts of the iris reflect changes in certain organs. The right iris shows the condition of the right side of the body, while the left iris reflects the left side.[3]

The iris is composed of densely structured, fine straight lines radiating from the pupil to the outer rim. A close grain indicates a strong inherited vitality and good recuperative powers in the case of temporary illness. If the fibers are loosely spread, the basic health is weak. I was able to see progress in my iris at every visit, especially in the area that was related to my lungs. It was exciting to see how real this was, and how what I ate affected my health—and my iris!

I was eating homemade cassava pizza at home while my friends were eating burgers and hotdogs. My friends marveled at my refrigerator when they came over. It was filled with healthy foods. I felt proud of my eating habits and was so grateful my mom cared so much to take me to a doctor that could actually make me better. I was medication free and in great health.

One of the most impactful things Dr. Norman taught me is that it's not good to drink beverages while having a meal. It is best to avoid beverages 15 minutes before you begin eating and wait an hour after that meal to begin drinking again in order to aid the digestion process. Being hydrated before a meal will help kick-start your metabolism, but drinking while eating makes it harder for your body to digest the meal. Drinking cold beverages while eating may be particularly harmful to the digestion process. Hot drinks, such as tea, are better.

I usually drink plenty of water throughout the whole day, but put my intake on hold especially during heavy meals like lunch. I'll take a sip of water if I'm thirsty during the meal, but won't gulp my drink away.

Naturopathic care during pregnancy.

Fast-forward 15 years. I was still a vegetarian, but I ate a bunch of junk that Dr. Norman would not be proud of. I lost my way a bit, and I wasn't in optimal health, although my asthma was pretty much under control and only surfaced about once a year during Christmas time.

It was my Pastor's wife, Carey, who encouraged me to try healthier foods again. She talked to me about the benefits of fish oil and coconut oil. I checked out my local health food store and all the memories of shopping healthy with my mom during my teens came back.

I thought I was on the fast track to optimal health and a healthy pregnancy when my asthma resurfaced after three months of pregnancy. I read that many women experience asthma during pregnancy in addition to allergies and other issues stemming from a compromised immune system. Even though I knew the OB community didn't have a problem with the use of an inhaler during pregnancy, I did. I wanted my baby to have the best possible start and health and I didn't want anything to be a roadblock to that process.

I mentioned my dilemma to my friend Leilani, and she recommended that I visit the naturopath that helped her get pregnant, Dr. Gisela Hernandez de Antuña. She found that the root cause of my asthma was low immunity, so she increased my immunity to improve my health and begin healing. I started my naturopathic treatment that first trimester with Bella and shortly after, my asthma was gone—again. I have not experienced an asthma attack since.

During my first visit, I was hopeful that Dr. Hernandez would help me get back on track just like Dr. Norman was able to do so many years ago. I called her office to make an appointment and was asked to bring the results of my most recent blood work. I was so excited the day I went to see her at her office in Aventura, FL. The staff was really nice. She welcomed me into her office, sat me down, and said, "You have allergies . . ." "Well, I have a runny nose here and there," I replied. "No, you ARE allergic," she replied in an I-am-not-asking-you-I-am-telling-you kind of way. I was in shock. How did she know? She said she could see it in my blood, and that we had to address that right away.

Dr. Hernandez checked my eyes using iridology during my first visit, just like Dr. Norman used to do. She also tested my muscles for strength and weakness. She then used a BioElectrical Impedance Measurement (BIM) machine that measures how the meridians (or electrical circuits) in your body relate to specific organs and systems. It is similar to an EKG or EEG machine, which are used to measure heart or brain function. The examination is performed by testing up to 60 acupressure points, which relate back to the meridians and their related organs, systems, or functions.[4] The great thing about the BIM is that it generates a report card that allows you to track your progress over time. Although feeling better was proof enough for me, it was cool to see how my health was improving in a report.

This assessment does not involve needles, only a stylus that is similar to a pen, which sends a very small and unnoticeable electrical current through each point. The computer system records your measurements and compares it to a database of over 1.5 million tests in order to identify the areas of your body that have moved outside the norm. The BIM then generates a report card with the functional status of all your meridians and their related organs, systems, and functions. You are able to see which ones are stressed, balanced, or weakened, and by how much. Lastly, the software helps the provider match the best supplements for your needs. The best match is the supplement that brings the unbalanced meridians back to balance.

Dr. Hernandez told me my immune system was very low while her assistant performed the assessment. She explained this was very normal during pregnancy, but assured me that we

would fix it. She then grabbed various supplements from her pantry to test on the BIM machine. Dr. Hernandez explained that everyone does not respond the same way to the same supplement. She placed the different supplements on a platform that was part of the BIM, one at a time, and retested the acupressure point. Some supplements were either too strong or too weak. She chose the supplement or combination of supplements that brought my acupressure points back to range.

The BIM assessment took about 40 minutes. Dr. Hernandez put together a list of supplements after checking all my acupressure points and testing all the supplements and protein powders. The first one I had to take—first thing in the morning—was liquid chlorophyll.

Chlorophyll is the green pigment in plants that harnesses the sun's energy in photosynthesis. The chlorophyll molecule is chemically similar to human blood, except its central atom is magnesium, whereas that of human blood is iron. This means that when ingested, liquid chlorophyll can actually help to do the job of hemoglobin. This is especially beneficial during pregnancy when hemoglobin levels are at a risk of running low.

Hemoglobin is so vital to the health of our blood—in fact, approximately 75% of our blood is hemoglobin. Taking liquid chlorophyll helps rebuild and replenish our red blood cells, boosting our energy and increasing our well being almost instantly.

I like the liquid chlorophyll by Nature's Sunshine. It has a nice and subtle minty taste and it isn't refined and highly processed (which kills the nutrients) or filled with sweeteners that suppress your immune system, like most other chlorophyll supplements.

I began taking one teaspoon with water upon waking up. After one month, Dr. Hernandez increased the dosage to 3 tablespoons taken throughout the day. I added a tablespoon to my water jug in the morning, then again at noon, and lastly in the afternoon. I made sure to finish all the water before refilling again to keep track of how much chlorophyll I was drinking.

My Pregnancy Diet Plan

Naturopathic treatment considers your personal biology and your personal physiology. Therefore, the supplements and diet are tailored to your genetics and seek to alter any adverse predispositions. Sometimes that means removing foods that are causing an imbalance and don't let our bodies function properly, in order to achieve optimal health.

This means that not everyone with the same disease has the same treatment or the same

cause. Every person is different, and a particular disease will manifest differently in different people. With that in mind, check out my personalized pregnancy diet plan **(Table 6.1)** as prescribed by my naturopath, Dr. Gisela Hernandez.

Fighting constipation with flaxseed.

Flaxseed water is a great way to fight constipation and aid your digestive process. Dr. Hernandez explained it is important to have a healthy digestive system because that is how

TABLE 6.1 SAMPLE OF PERSONALIZED PREGNANCY DIET PLAN

	Supplement	Drink	Option 1	Option 2	Option 3
First thing in the morning:	Liquid Chlorophyll by Nature's Sunshine	Drink 8 oz. of water mixed with one teaspoon of liquid chlorophyll.			
Breakfast:	1 Proprenatal Complex (prenatal vitamin) 2 Immuplex by Standard Process (to increase immunity) 2 Folate (for baby's nervous development)	Alfalfa tea	Protein shake: 1 scoop of i5 protein powder ADD all the following: 1/4 Teaspoon of igG2000DF (to increase immunity) 1 teaspoon bee propolis (to increase immunity) 1 teaspoon royal jelly (to increase immunity) 1 teaspoon wheat germ (for iron) 1 tablespoon Lecithin Granules (Baby's brain development)	Hot cereal: oat bran, amaranth, rice bran, or spelt (Tip: presoak cereal overnight) Mix in 2 tablespoons of protein powder (i5) Add papaya, strawberries, pineapple, or dried fruits (one at a time) Only add sweetener after cooking or reheating Or add seeds and nuts: Sesame, walnuts, almonds, or grated coconut	Egg white omelet with vegetables
Lunch	Supplements Lunch: 1 Proprenatal, 2 Immuplex	Alfalfa tea, raspberry tea, ginger tea, GI Protect Juice	Fish or veggie burger (low in soy) Good carbs: potato, pumpkin, sweet potato Grains: tabouli, hummus, quinoa Rice: golden rose, wild rice Any beans	Any soups	Quinoa noodles or pasta, rice noodles or pasta, brown rice pasta, or spelt pasta

TABLE 6.1 CONT'D...

	Supplement	Drink	Option 1	Option 2	Option 3
Afternoon Snack			Protein shake: 1 scoop of i5 protein powder ADD all the following: 1/4 teaspoon of igG2000DF (to increase immunity) 1 teaspoon bee propolis (to increase immunity) 1 teaspoon royal jelly (to increase immunity) 1 teaspoon wheat germ (for iron) 1 tablespoon Lecithin Granules (for baby's brain development)		
Dinner		Alfalfa tea, raspberry tea, ginger tea, GI Protect Juice	Fish or veggie burger (low in soy) Good carbs: potato, pumpkin, sweet potato Grains: tabouli, hummus, quinoa Rice: golden rose, wild rice Any beans	Any soups	Quinoa noodles or pasta, rice noodles or pasta, brown rice pasta, or spelt pasta
Bedtime		6 oz. flaxseed water (see preparation below)			

No: Wheat.

Avoid: Preservatives (canned or frozen foods), fried foods, refined flour, pasteurized dairy, and processed foods.

Maybe: Raw dairy is healthier (homogenized and pasteurization kills enzymes) but whether it is beneficial or not depends on the person. If you are predisposed and cannot metabolize, you can generate phlegm and become irritated. A person with allergies may have an adverse reaction even when milk is consumed raw.

we absorb the nutrients from the foods we eat and how our baby is going to be nourished as well. If we are not nourished, our baby won't be either.

Drink six ounces of flax seed water before bedtime and drink enough water throughout the day. Flaxseed is rich in fiber, which helps cleanse the colon of toxins and metabolic waste. You will love this if you suffer from constipation!

Preparation: Soak flaxseed in water for at least 8 hours. Strain them and drink the liquid only, which will become slimy. You can save the flax and add it to soups, salad dressings, or smoothies. You can prepare flaxseed water ahead of time in a large quantity and keep it refrigerated for later use. The ratio is 2:1 ounces of water to teaspoons of flax. I make enough for 4 days at a time, so I fill a jug will 24 ounces of water and 12 teaspoons of flax. It tastes better cold, so keep it refrigerated.

Each trimester brought a change. I kept the same diet throughout my entire pregnancy, but made a few changes to the supplements.

During the second trimester, I increased the liquid chlorophyll to 3 tablespoons throughout the day. I was given the option to switch to Immune Stimulator instead of Immuplex (2 at breakfast, 2 at lunch, and 1 at dinner) and I took GI Protect (1 scoop twice a day with water).

During the third trimester, I took a prenatal at breakfast <u>and</u> lunch. I also took Immuplex (2 at breakfast, 2 at lunch) and 2 Inositol (if I didn't have an i5 protein shake in the afternoon to maintain my sugar levels). I supplemented throughout the day with 16 ounces of homemade vegetable juice (such as carrot, beets with leaves, spinach, celery, green chard, cucumber, kale, and broccoli), took calcium plus vitamin D (2 at dinner and 2 at bedtime), and started taking 5-W five weeks before my due date (2 at breakfast, 2 at lunch, 2 at dinner). This is a natural supplement that helps women dilate for birth.

Action Step: Call a naturopath and tell them you need help coming up with a pregnancy diet. Ask for the consultation fee and have an established budget for supplements prior to the visit. Naturopathic care is yet to be covered by most insurance, but you'll be surprised how affordable it is compared to some conventional medicine treatments.

My budget for the visit is: _____

My budget for supplements is: _____

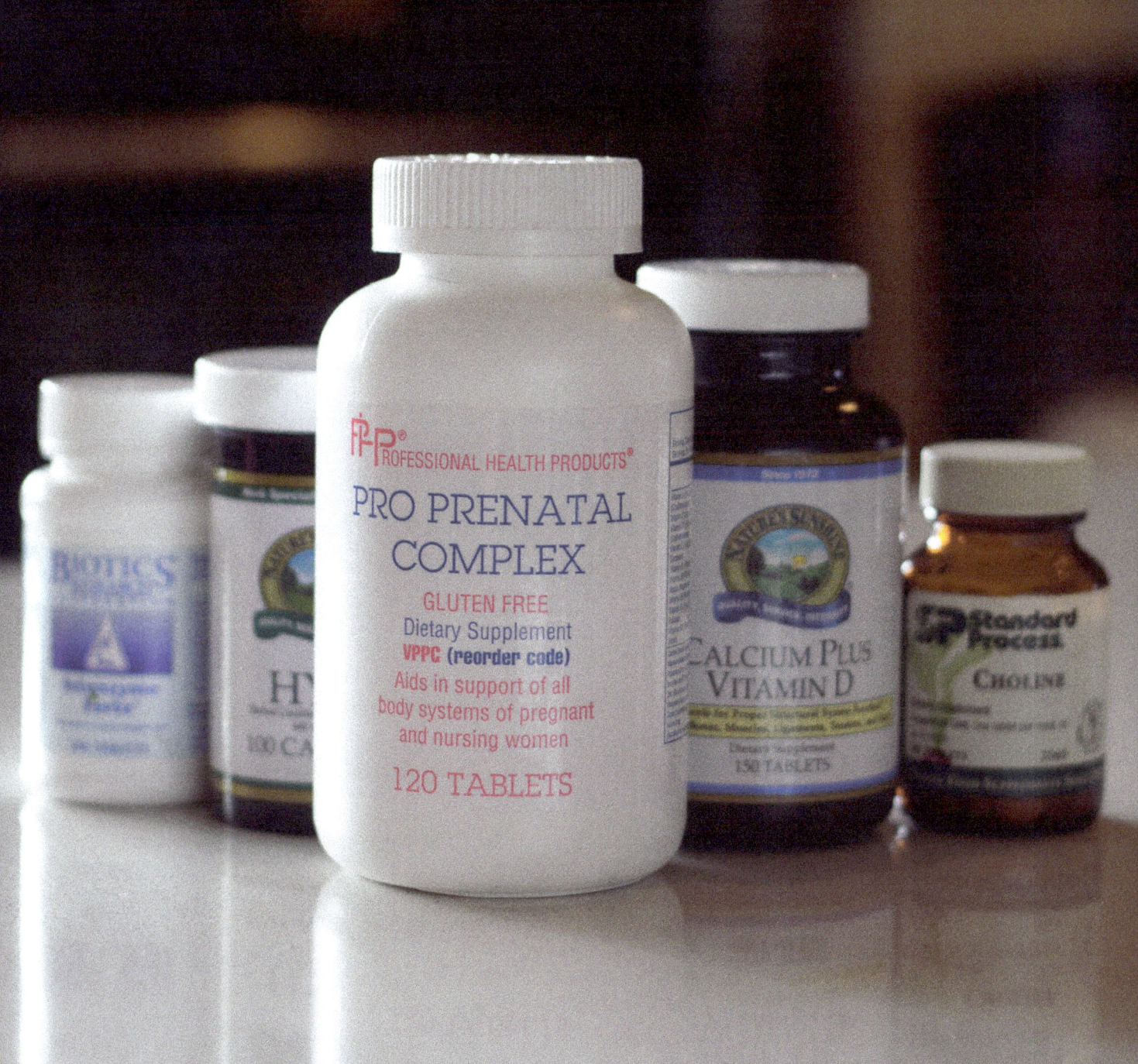

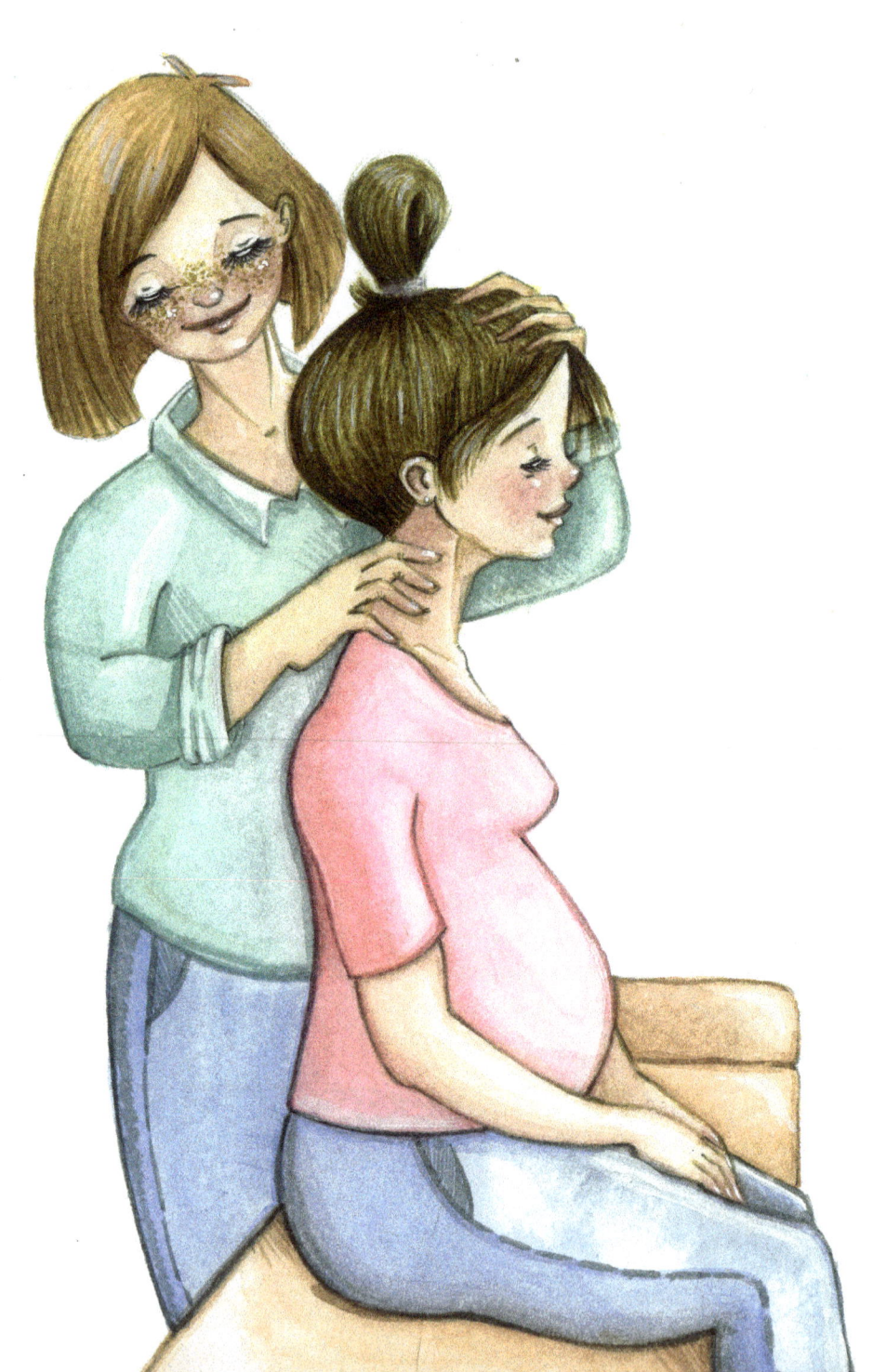

CHAPTER 7

How Chiropractic Changed My Life

It was the first day of October, 2010, and I had just dropped off my son, John, at his girlfriend's house when a 53' truck drove into the back of my small car. I remember hitting the breaks with all of my strength as if that could stop my car from hitting the car in front of me. The truck pushed my car down the road until the driver realized what was happening. Because the truck was missing the mirror that reflects what is directly in front of it, the driver didn't see my car (which was below his line of vision) when the light turned green. He just went on as if there was only space between him and the car in front of me. Thankfully, the car in front of me drove away and avoided my hit.

I wasn't alone in the car. My daughter, Abi, was riding in the front passenger seat and her brother, Guillermo, was in his car seat in the back. Thankfully, she just experienced a few headaches that eventually went away, and Guillermo had fun being the center of attention at the urgent care unit that we went to. I had a lot of pressure in my lower back and near my shoulder, which became worse the next day. I took the pain medication that I was given at the urgent care center, but it was awful. Yes, it took away the pain, but it also took away my energy and zeal. I slept the whole day while my kids were in school. The pain came back the next day. Since I knew the pain medication would not heal my injury, and I was preheating for pregnancy, I decided to put up with the pain without it. I had a family to attend to and could not afford its side effects.

I went to an orthopedic surgeon who immediately prescribed an MRI and the results showed two herniated discs. Fortunately, I wasn't a candidate for surgery, which meant that the orthopedic surgeon couldn't do anything but dismiss me. I would just have to "manage the pain." I went to physical therapy, but I didn't feel any improvement and stopped going altogether when JC and I started trying to conceive because I wanted to avoid any unnecessary ultrasounds. Be mindful of such diagnostic tests while you are pregnant because x-rays give off cancer-causing radiation.

Pregnant and In Pain

I first noticed my lower back pain becoming sharp and very bothersome at around my third month of pregnancy. It seemed like the baby was pushing into the herniated disc in my lower back as she was growing. I read that this was normal, so I was coping with the back pain but was not enjoying my pregnancy very much as a result.

Getting my Back on Track

I was about four months pregnant when my friend, Samantha C., told me that she went to a chiropractor with her husband, Ivan, and noticed that they treated pregnant women. She encouraged me to go check it out and see if they could help me with my back pain. I was initially skeptical. I'd "heard" that chiropractors were bad and that I should never go to one, but I also felt hopeful. If the conventional route couldn't do anything for me, maybe this would. I became open-minded and began doing research on chiropractic and pregnancy in my desperation for a solution to my pain. Not only did I find out that it was beneficial, but most importantly, it was safe.

I made an appointment and drove many miles to get to their office. Every mile was worth it because that's how I met my friends Dr. Joe Coffman and his wife Dr. Lisa. Their office was very welcoming, very different from any other medical office that I had been to. The staff was very friendly and it felt right to be there. I was given literature on chiropractic care to read while I waited. The waiting area had books and toys for children.

I first met with Dr. Joe. He performed some tests to assess my spine and nervous system, checked my posture, and carefully examined the results of my MRI because he couldn't take any x-rays due to my pregnancy. He further explained chiropractic care and how it could help me, the baby, and the upcoming delivery. When I asked him if he could permanently

take the pain away, he said that he couldn't do anything; he explained my body was the one that had the ability to heal from anything and that they were just going to help my body work and heal the way it was intended to. He said that by working to restore the normal motion and alignment in my spine, the nervous system would function at its best, which would give my body and my baby the best chance at not only permanent pain relief but optimal health. I was convinced! I was so happy that someone finally explained health in a way that made sense.

He further explained chiropractic in a very simple way:

As you may know, chiropractors specialize in the spine, just like cardiologists work with the heart. The spine has two primary functions. One, it supports you, and keeps you upright. The way your spine supports you is called your posture. Two, and most importantly, it's the only thing that surrounds and protects your spinal cord.

A healthy spinal cord is essential to your overall health. Your brain controls all the functions of your body. It does this by sending electrical energy down your spinal cord. Your spinal cord is like a river, carrying life energy from your brain, through your spine to all the vital organs and tissues of your body. Each and every organ (like your reproductive organs) is totally dependent on that energy to keep you alive and healthy. And as soon as you conceive you'll essentially have another 'organ,' your baby, and he or she will be totally dependent on that neurological energy to develop, grow, and thrive.

Because of different stresses in your life—some sudden, and some over time—the bones in your spine shift out of place. When these shifts occur, they disrupt the normal nervous system function. It's like a dimmer light switch on a wall. The energy gets turned down, it can't get through the nerves to your organs (and baby) properly, and the organs at the end of those nerves immediately weaken, begin to malfunction, develop conditions and diseases, and degenerate.

These misalignments will also weaken the rest of the structure of your spine and distort your posture. When your posture weakens and distorts, it causes tension on your spinal cord. When your spinal cord is under stress, it cannot properly move energy through the spine to all the vital organs of your body (and baby). When your organs don't get the vital energy they need, your overall health is in severe distress, significantly increasing your likelihood of developing serious degenerative diseases.

Now this is really important: most postural distortions and misalignments (subluxations) don't even cause any pain. And many times there is no pain in the early stages of organ disease. By the time you're in pain, your nerves are inflamed, and your body is in a crisis. So, if you're experiencing lower back pain, that means the nerves exiting your lower spine are inflamed, your body isn't getting energy through them well, and the organs at the end of those nerves are also being affected. Guess where else the nerves of the lower spine supply neurological energy? That's right, your baby!

One of the staff members then taught me "warm-up" exercises to prepare me for the adjustment. These exercises helped restore and keep my spinal discs hydrated. They also helped circulate cerebral spinal fluid (CSF). CSF is the fluid that flows around the brain and spinal cord carrying nutrients and helping to transmit impulses. These warm-ups were very important to get the best results from my adjustments.

After I finished the exercises, it was time for my first adjustment. I swiped my entry card, just like at the gym, and was called to one of their tables. I was quite nervous, but put on my best poker face. The first adjustment was facing down, so Dr. Joe modified the table so that my growing belly was comfortable. I could only hear and feel the table moving as he adjusted my lower back. That wasn't so bad, I thought. I then rolled over and he adjusted my middle back with what seemed like a big hug. This is when I first heard the famous popping sound that your bones make when they are adjusted. (I say popping because cracking is a bad word in chiropractic.) It felt like a great release. Dr. Joe explained to me that the noise I was hearing and feeling was merely air in the joints. Lastly, he placed his hand on my neck to adjust it. I tried to relax, but I was so nervous about this one. I, like so many others, was scared because

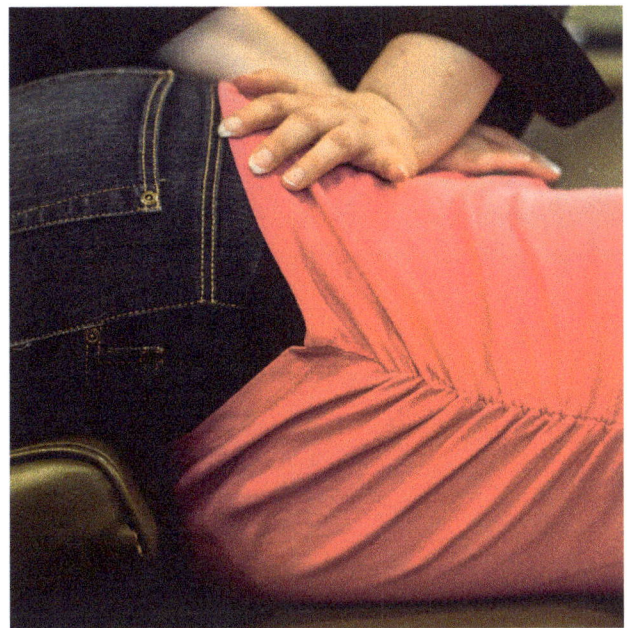

I have watched a few movies where someone gets killed by having the neck snapped, and just the thought of someone holding my neck freaked me out. But Dr. Joe adjusted me before I could think about it too much—and it felt great! They had me perform specific postural movements after the adjustment to help extend the benefits of the adjustment and correct my spinal alignment.

This was my experience as a patient, but my doctors are very specific about tailoring chiropractic care to what's best for the individual. I have come to realize how very unique and different their care is! Not all doctors are the same.

I encourage you to look for one that is right for you. Interview a few of them before you decide on one that you feel is the most qualified and one who you feel comfortable with.

Making Regular Visits

I was completely pain free after just a few weeks! Chiropractic treatment eliminated my back pain and helped me become a healthier person. Dr. Joe encouraged me to work out during pregnancy, and I was enjoying my daily aerobic or prenatal yoga video. I also had a lot of energy and was enjoying my pregnancy more than I ever imagined I would.

I became more knowledgeable about the different systems of the body during my visits to the chiropractor. I learned that a healthy spine results in a healthy body and mind, that God gave us an immune system to protect our bodies, and our immune system must be healthy for us to stay healthy. As Dr. Joe explained, chiropractic care helps me maintain a healthy immune system by ensuring that my brain can send the chemicals that my body needs in order to heal. My body can work adequately and can innately protect itself when it is free from subluxations.

Stress, a workout or sports injury, carrying a heavy box, sleeping in a bad position, being sick, poor eating habits, pregnancy, and childbirth, are a few of the things that can cause subluxations. The best way to be free of subluxations is to visit a chiropractor regularly. Your visits can range from three times per week to bi-weekly depending on your severity and stress levels. The key is to commit to an adjustment schedule that is right for your body. If you only go to the gym once, whenever your jeans feel tight, you wouldn't see much change. I get adjusted regularly—just like I exercise regularly. It's part of my lifestyle.

I don't think that I would have ever gone to a chiropractor if it weren't for my injury. I am grateful that God used that car accident to introduce me to chiropractic. The car accident that led me to Drs. Coffman led me to a healthy pregnancy and natural childbirth. I have learned so much from Dr. Joe and Dr. Lisa. I am healthier because my body is working as God designed it to be. God makes everything work for our well-being.

The Matos Family

There was another family that also got adjusted regularly, the Matos family. Niki (the wife) and Jose (her husband) had two little ones, Genesis and Isaac. Genesis was just a newborn and Isaac was a toddler. I remember the day I met them and learned their newborn baby would also get adjusted. I was fascinated and asked if I could see the adjustment. It was a beautiful sight. The infant adjustment was soft and very gentle. Niki told me that Genesis took the best naps right after an adjustment.

Niki shared her experiences about birth and motherhood with me as we continued bumping into each other at the chiropractor. She answered all of my questions related to pregnancy, birth, and caring for a baby. She described how she didn't know about chiropractic during her first pregnancy (with Isaac) and how she was always tired and in pain. She contrasted it to her pregnancy with Genesis when she was getting adjusted regularly, and shared she was pain-free and felt very energetic even toward the end of her pregnancy. She also told me about how helpful it was for Dr. Lisa to assist her during her labor with Genesis.

I thought that was all so cool. I wondered if Dr. Lisa could help manage my pain with her adjustments and pressure points because I wanted a natural birth. I didn't know how much Dr. Lisa would charge for something like this, so I asked Niki before even approaching her. She nodded and said, "Nothing." I was surprised and thought that maybe it was something Dr. Lisa did for her because they were friends. I asked Dr. Lisa directly after I got adjusted, and she told me she would be honored to be with me during my labor and that she did that for her patients. I was amazed she would do that out

of the kindness of her heart—that she would be willing to wake up in the middle of the night to assist me in Bella's birth.

The Doctor that Led Me to My Midwife

Dr. Lisa asked me about how the baby and I were doing every time that she adjusted me. I could tell she cared about her patients.

One day Dr. Lisa asked me about my birth plan. I told her I wanted a natural birth. She then asked me if I would consider a home birth and suggested that I watch a documentary called *The Business of Being Born*, and even let me borrow her copy.

Having a home birth became a very real option in my birth plan after watching the documentary. Dr. Lisa was very excited to learn that I was open to it and took it upon herself to interview several midwives for me, and ultimately gave me a flyer to The Miami Midwife, Sheila Simms Watson; I kept the flyer even though I was afraid to call her. After Dr. Lisa asked me a couple of times if I had called Sheila (I hadn't), I finally decided to call her. After meeting her, I was confident she would be my midwife.

I wish more doctors would take the time to educate their patients on natural birthing and home births as a real alternative.

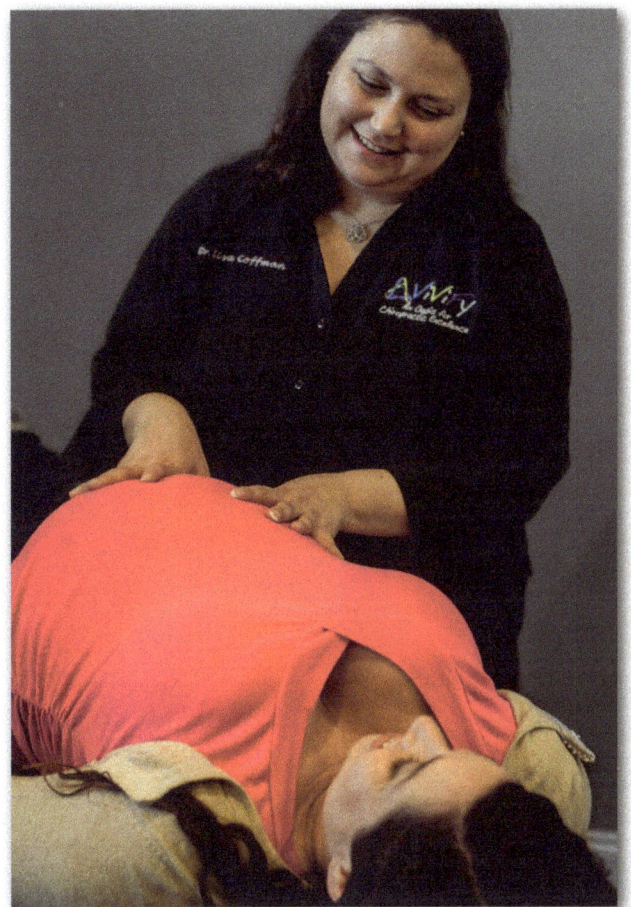

DR. LISA WITH SAMANTHA L.

The Webster Technique

Dr. Lisa checked to see how Bella was positioned further along in my pregnancy. We noticed that Bella was breech, and Sheila later confirmed it. Dr. Lisa told me it was going to be fine and that she knew a technique developed by Larry Webster, D.C., which could allow more

Dr. Joe Coffman describes the Webster technique, like this:

> *In a nutshell: As the sacrum and pelvis shifts out of its normal position, it does three things: pulls on the muscles and ligaments, closing off the birth canal; distorts the round ligaments of the uterus increasing tension; and irritates the nerves going to the uterus. Those three things reduce the space for the baby to get into the optimal position, head down, and engage the cervix. If left uncorrected, it can result in a breech baby or difficult labor. The Webster's technique helps to restore normal biomechanics of the pelvis, allow the uterus to relax, and give more room for the baby to get into the best position for birth. That's why moms that get adjusted throughout their pregnancy seem to have greater comfort, less interventions, and easier births.*

room for Bella to turn. During Dr. Webster's career of working with over 1,000 pregnant moms, he reported that over 90% of the babies optimized their positioning in utero when the mother received this sacral adjustment. So, I alternated between my normal adjustment and the Webster technique, and Bella eventually turned.

Thomas D'amico, D.C., a pediatric chiropractor in Davie, Florida, says that using Dr. Webster's technique for breech babies allows them to get into the proper position 99% of the time in his practice. Dr. D'amico clarifies that this technique is not to be confused with the external cephalic version performed by an obstetrician, by which babies are externally moved by putting pressure on the mother's womb. He says that technique can actually be very hurtful to the mother and damaging to the baby. The external cephalic version has a success rate of only 58%.[1] Visit *www.icpa4kids*.org to find a list of doctors with a special interest and training in caring for pregnant mothers, infants, and children, and to find a chiropractor who is trained in the Webster Technique.

How to Choose a Good Chiropractor

Table 7.1 includes a questionnaire that Drs. Coffman developed to help you find a good chiropractor.

TABLE 7.1: CHIROPRACTOR INTERVIEW QUESTIONS

Question	Considerations
What is your primary technique?	A "diversified" approach is not too impressive, as that is a very basic mishmash that has very few measures of analysis. Look for a place that has a specific system for determining adjustments (when to adjust, when not to adjust, what to adjust, and what to do once the adjustment has been made). A handful of techniques with a good system of analysis are: Activator, Atlas Orthogonal, Chiropractic BioPhysics (CBP), Kale, NUCCA, Pettibon, and Torque Release Technique.
What percentage of your practice are kids?	They should know the percentage. 40% is a great benchmark, but anything above 25% is good.
What's your opinion on therapies such as ultrasound and electric stimulation?	These therapies are forms of pain management, rather than chiropractic. Ideally, your chiropractor will not use pain therapies at all.
Do you conduct re-exams?	A good chiropractor conducts re-exams to evaluate their clinical outcomes and determine if they need to modify your care in order to achieve optimal results.
What type of objective criteria do you use to determine that the spine and nervous system are functioning better?	Examples of reliable objective criteria are: X-rays, digital posture, digital muscle testing, digital range of motion, Thermography, Surface ElectroMyoGraphy (SEMG), and Heart Rate Variability.

Bella's Birth and the First Months

I started having contractions and felt water running down my leg on my way to the bathroom on September 16, 2011 at 4:05 AM. "Babe, wake up! I think my water broke!" I told my husband JC with excitement. Dr. Lisa told me that I could call her at any point in my labor when I wanted her to come over. I called her to give her a heads up and told her I would call her once the contractions got stronger. We called her at about 6:30 AM, and she drove over from her apartment in Miami Beach to be with me.

Dr. Lisa performed a few adjustments that felt good during labor. She released my abdominal muscles by putting pressure on a point behind my thigh when my contractions got really intense. She also checked that my pelvis was aligned so that Bella could easily descend. She put cold compresses on my head so I could refresh and get ready to push once we realized that Bella was right there. She was my doula, and she was there the moment that Bella said hello to the world. She even heated up soup for me afterwards. She checked and adjusted Bella and me about an hour after Bella was born.

Dr. Lisa came to my house and adjusted us during those first couple of months. Those first weeks were so tough, but she was there. I had to overcome struggles during breastfeeding, but she was there. That's how we became friends.

The Pubic Bone Adjustment and Mila's Birth

I was receiving chiropractic care even before I conceived Mila. Mila's pregnancy was so easy-going that I had no symptoms of being pregnant. Zero. I had lots of energy. Unlike with Bella's pregnancy, where my asthma resurfaced before I began chiropractic care, I was in perfect health. I experienced lower back pain with Bella before beginning chiropractic care. With Mila, I got adjusted whenever I got a little sore, and that was it. The pain just went away. I was truly in optimal health.

But something was off at 39 weeks. Even though Sheila was certain that Mila could be born at any time, and I was experiencing Braxton-Hicks for a while, I would not go into labor. I was having pre-labor contractions on and off since Thursday morning. It was now Monday and nothing was happening. I was at Dr. Lisa's office and told her about my irregular contractions, and she immediately checked my pubic bone.

Dr. Lisa explained that your pelvis might shift slightly as it expands to make room for the baby. This causes the pubic bone to be uneven and makes it difficult for the baby to make her way through the pelvis and out. She then asked me to walk around for 5-10 minutes after she adjusted it. That's when I felt Mila fit into place. I literally felt her descend until her head was right on my pubic bone. I went into labor that same night.

Mila's birth was so quick that our midwife could not even make it on time. Dr. Lisa arrived right after I gave birth. She checked and adjusted Mila a few of hours after she was born and she adjusted me the next day.

Evelyn

My friend Evelyn was getting adjusted by a chiropractor throughout her pregnancy. I told her how the pubic bone adjustment was very beneficial to me and encouraged her to make sure that hers was aligned for birth. Her chiropractor hadn't performed it when one day, at 39 weeks, she began having contractions. Her contractions came regularly, but then slowed down at times. She had these inconsistent contractions all day Saturday. It was now Sunday, and Evelyn was still not progressing. I called Dr. Lisa and asked her if she would be willing to check Evelyn. Their office was closed, but I was hopeful she would be willing to help us.

Dr. Lisa came over and checked Evelyn. She quickly realized that Evelyn's pubic bone was extremely misaligned and that she needed to adjust her. It was likely that Evelyn would be in labor for hours and end up with a C-section because her baby wouldn't be able to fit through the pelvis without an adjustment.

After Dr. Lisa adjusted Evelyn, she shared some pain management tips with George, Evelyn's

husband. Evelyn went into labor that night and their baby, Sarah, was born the next morning. Evelyn was her doctor's only patient to birth vaginally that day. The rest were C-sections.

Samantha C

My friend, Samantha C., was the very first person to ever talk to me about home births and told me about Drs. Coffman.

I remember her trying to birth at home with her first-born, Noah. She was in labor for 24 hours before they decided to go to the hospital instead. Samantha was very supportive and excited for me when I decided to opt for a home birth. She knew I was going to the chiropractor and told me how beneficial it would have been for her to have chiropractic care in preparation for her pregnancy because managing her back pain was the toughest thing for her during labor.

Samantha decided to give home birthing another shot when she got pregnant again. This time, however, she was going to make sure she took care of her back first. So, she began chiropractic care and made sure to ask Dr. Lisa for her invaluable support during birth.

I was with Samantha the night she went into labor. I saw her during those first few hours and was so proud of her as she breathed through her contractions. I left, Dr. Lisa arrived, and Elijah was born two hours later. It is the hardest thing she has ever done, but she did it! Samantha experienced her much desired, long-awaited, natural home birth. The birth of her dreams! And we were all so proud of her.

Action Step: Call a chiropractor and ask about going for a consultation. Look for a chiropractor that will create a treatment plan where you can go a couple of times a week to get checked and adjusted during pregnancy.

I will visit, call, or get more information on these chiropractors: _____

_____

_____

My monthly budget for the chiropractor is: _____

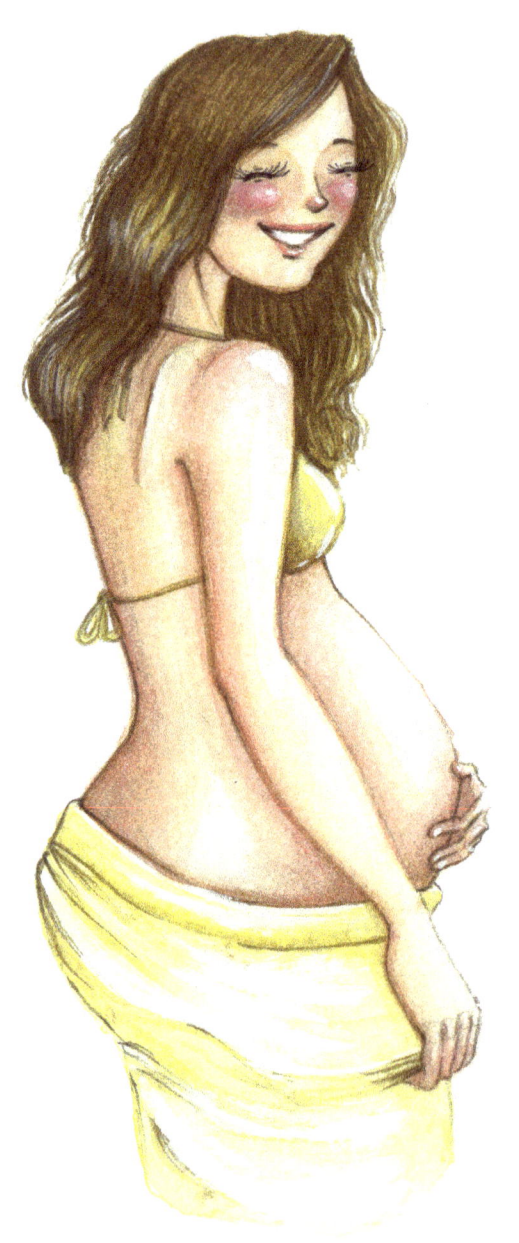

CHAPTER 8

Enjoying Pregnancy

I loved being pregnant! Having my baby in my womb made me feel more valuable and precious than ever. I received more compliments while I was pregnant than I ever had before. I heard about how radiant my skin was and how energized and healthy I looked. Not only was this a result of pregnancy hormones, but also a result of my diligence in making sure to care for my body during each stage. You have a baby that is literally competing with you for resources when you are pregnant. This is why it makes such a difference to pay extra attention to your body throughout the whole way.

Remember that regular exercise, good nutrition, and naturopathic and chiropractic care are important fundamentals that make a huge positive impact on your health and your baby. Part One of this chapter shares a few ways to complement those fundamentals with some "me" time. In Part Two, I share ways to bond with your baby during pregnancy so you can establish the foundation of your future relationship. Part Three covers changes to your body and baby by trimester. And in Part Four we talk about sex. Get ready to love being pregnant!

Part One: Me Time

Most of us are rarely without anything to do. We love to be busy and accomplish goals. This is why I want you to add some "me" time to your to do list. This time is an investment in your body. You will thank me for it later.

Prevent stretch marks. Hydrating your skin with natural oils like almond oil, coconut oil, and olive oil will increase its elasticity so that you don't get stretch marks as your baby grows. If you began hydrating during preheating, you will have an advantage.

Some people believe it doesn't matter if you use creams or not because you will or will not get stretch marks depending on your skin type. They believe you are basically predetermined. I disagree. Your diet, how much you eat, and the size of your baby affect your odds of getting stretch marks.

Almond oil is my favorite body oil and I practically bathed in it while I was pregnant. However, I alternated oils weekly or biweekly so that my skin didn't get used to one and therefore maximized the effect of the oils. I made it a point to apply the oil all over my body, but made sure to emphasize the growing areas like the breasts, belly, and hips. I did this after every shower and whenever else I remembered. My skin looked radiant throughout both of my pregnancies, but most importantly, I didn't get any stretch marks.

Choose all-natural face and body soaps. Popular soaps contain ingredients that are harsh and may even be toxic to your body. My philosophy is to watch out for ingredients that would be toxic if ingested. If you are likely to die from drinking it, then you shouldn't be putting it on your skin.

Organic and alkaline chemicals can soften the keratin cells on the skin and pass through this layer to the dermis, where they are able to enter the veins and the blood stream. Chemicals can also enter through cuts, punctures, or scrapes on the skin since these are breaks in the protective layer.[1] You should also make sure that your soaps are as safe and natural as possible because taking a hot shower opens up your skin pores and vaporizes 70 to 90% of the chemicals present and you can even inhale them into your lungs.

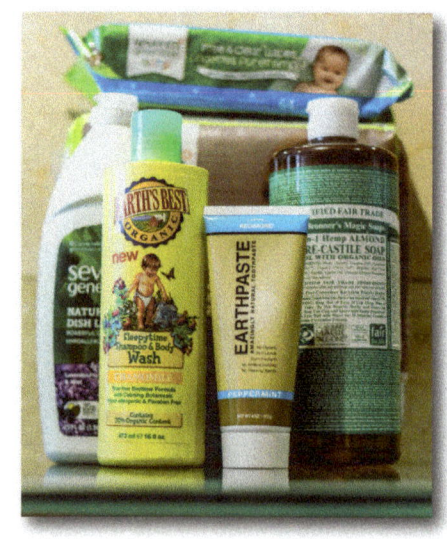

Look for the genuine USDA Organic seal when buying products. I recommend checking out the Environmental Working Group's Skin Deep Cosmetic Safety Database[2] or another website called GoodGuide[3] to see how your products rate for safety. I like Kiss My Face's Whenever Shampoo (about $11) and Dr. Bronner's Lavender and Almond Body Soaps (32 fl. oz. about $16). Make sure you hydrate with natural oils following your bath, since the soap cleanses the oils from your skin.

Be sure to avoid these seven ingredients when buying soaps: Sodium Lauryl/Laureth Sulfate (SLS/SLES), Dioxane, Parabens, Propylene Glycol, Diethanolamine or DEA, Fragrance Toluene, and Triclosan. See **Table 8.1** for more information on them.[4]

TABLE 8.1 SEVEN INGREDIENTS TO AVOID

	Description	Tips & Warnings
Sodium Lauryl/Laureth Sulfate (SLS/SLES)	SLS is rated by the Environmental Working Group's (EWG) Skin Deep Cosmetics Database as a "moderate hazard." SLS breaks down the skin's moisture barrier, easily penetrates the skin, and allows other chemicals to penetrate by increasing skin permeability by approximately 100-fold.	• Combined with other chemicals, SLS becomes a "nitrosamine," a potent class of carcinogen. • Research studies have linked SLS to skin and eye irritation, organ toxicity, reproductive and developmental toxicity, endocrine disruption, neurotoxicity, cellular changes, possible mutations, and cancer.
Dioxane	Common in a wide range of products as part of PEG, Polysorbates, Laureth, and ethoxylated alcohols. These compounds are usually contaminated with high concentrations of highly volatile 1,4-dioxane which is easily absorbed through the skin. This "probable carcinogen to humans" substance has received a "high hazard" rating from EWG's Skin Deep and is especially toxic to your brain, central nervous system, kidneys, and liver.	• A synthetic derivative of coconut, watch for misleading language on labels stating "comes from coconut." • Avoid any product with indications of ethoxylation, which include: "myreth," "oleth," "laureth," "ceteareth," any other "eth," "PEG," "polyethylene," "polyethylene glycol," "polyoxyethylene," or "oxynol."
Propylene Glycol	A common ingredient in personal care products.	• It has been shown to cause dermatitis, kidney or liver abnormalities, and may inhibit skin cell growth or cause skin irritation. It is also found in engine coolants, antifreeze, rubber cleaners, adhesives, and paints and varnishes.
Diethanolamine or DEA	A common ingredient in personal care products.	• DEA readily reacts with nitrite preservatives and contaminants to create nitrosodiethanolamine (NDEA), a known and potent carcinogen. • DEA also appears to block absorption of the nutrient choline, which is vital to brain development.
Toluene	Fragrance Toluene, made from petroleum or coal tar, is found in most synthetic fragrances.	• Chronic exposure is linked to anemia, lowered blood cell count, liver or kidney damage, and may affect a developing fetus. Synthetic fragrances can also be drying and irritating to your skin.

Taking warm baths. Warm baths are very soothing and helpful during pregnancy. They can certainly help relax those pelvic muscles that are stretching as the baby grows. Make sure the water is not so hot that your skin becomes red. If it is, then it is also too hot for your baby. I liked using Vitamin C tablets by Vitashower (the company that makes my shower filter) to neutralize the chlorine in the water and Lavender Oil for a relaxing scent.

Taking care of your teeth. Your changing hormones during pregnancy affect your gums. Visiting the dentist during your pregnancy will help you avoid cavities and pregnancy gingivitis. The hormonal changes during pregnancy may exaggerate the gum tissue's response to plaque and bacterial toxins, resulting in red, swollen, and bleeding gums. You can prevent this by effectively brushing your teeth, flossing, and having a cleaning during each trimester.

Tooth decay and tooth sensitivity may also occur during pregnancy as a result of sickness during the first trimester and craving acidic foods. This erodes the enamel, the outer layer of your teeth. Eating healthy will help keep your teeth strong. Your body absorbs calcium during pregnancy to form your baby's bones, so it is important to consume calcium-rich foods or take a good calcium supplement. I recommend Nature's Sunshine Calcium plus Vitamin D.

I also advise that you check the ingredients in your current toothpaste. Many popular toothpastes contain harmful ingredients, but we don't even check the label because we trust the brand. Make sure your toothpaste does not contain these harsh but common ingredients: Sodium Fluoride, Triclosan, Sodium Lauryl Sulfate, Propylene Glycol, and DEA.[5]

My favorite toothpaste is Xyli-White by Now Foods (about $3) and I've been using it for years. Earth's Paste (about $5) is another good option. They are both effective and don't contain harmful ingredients. Toms of Maine has a great mouthwash that JC likes. I like rinsing with water and sea salt.

Preparing your perineum. The perineum is the delicate area between the anus and the vagina. Tears to the perineum are common during childbirth, especially with the first child. However, you can prevent tears by properly caring for your perineum during pregnancy.

I applied natural oils, such as almond oil, coconut oil, and olive oil to this area starting at 35 weeks of pregnancy during both pregnancies. My first labor resulted in just a couple minor splints that did not require stitches. However, those splints were so painful whenever I had to use the bathroom after delivering that I made sure I did squats (even during labor) the second time so I wouldn't tear.

Some practitioners like to perform episiotomies, a surgical cut in the muscular perineum made just before delivery to enlarge the vaginal opening, but many agree that it is best to tear naturally. Research shows that women with a spontaneous tear generally recover in the same or less time and often with fewer complications than those who have an episiotomy.[6]

Kegel exercises can also help prevent tears during delivery because you learn how to relax your pelvic floor muscles.[7] They consist of tightening and relaxing your pelvic floor muscles. You can begin doing Kegels the moment you find out you are pregnant. The cool thing about Kegels is that you can do them anywhere very discretely. This helpful exercise requires very little but the key is remembering to do it throughout the day. Seeing my growing belly served as a good reminder to me, but my friend Samantha C. had little stickers that said "Kegels" and she would stick them on her things as reminders.

In addition, birthing in water or applying warm compresses to the perineum will increase blood flow to the area and increase the flexibility of the tissues. My friend, Samantha L., had her first water birth experience with her third child. This was her biggest baby of all and the only one that didn't cause tear to her perineum.

Prenatal massages. I enjoyed prenatal massages during both of my pregnancies—twice with Bella and once with Mila. Most places will only do prenatal massages starting at 12 weeks of pregnancy, when you are less at risk of complications, and up to 36 weeks of pregnancy, when you are not at risk of going into labor.

Facials. Cleansing your face from toxins can be very beneficial during pregnancy when outbreaks tend to happen. Make sure to let your esthetician know you are pregnant and choose a place that is careful about the ingredients in their products. A facial is a nice treat that you can do every trimester to feel rejuvenated.

Caring for your feet. It is common for your feet to get swollen during pregnancy, especially the end. I recommend you wear comfortable sneakers as much as possible during pregnancy. I got a manicure and pedicure about once a month after my first trimester and that helped me feel better about myself. Avoid salons with strong smells. I did my own manicures at home many times for that reason. You can also find a nail technician that comes to you. Avoid getting your ankles massaged, since this may trigger premature contractions.

Waxing. I waxed every month during pregnancy and made sure I had my bikini area done close to my due date. There are mixed positions about waxing down under, but whatever position you choose, make sure to keep the area clean to avoid infections during pregnancy that may lead to the uncomfortable use of IV antibiotics, which may even be used during labor.

Looking great. Looking great during pregnancy will make you feel good as well. I wore nice workout clothes most of the time I was at home or out and about. This was helpful in two ways: I was comfortable and I could easily decide to work out because I was already dressed. This was particularly easy during my first pregnancy, but also during my second one when having a toddler made any activity, such as a visit to the park or a stroll around the neighborhood, a potential workout.

How to afford safe and healthy products for your "me" time. I began saving lots of money on my groceries when I subscribed to Amazon Mom. I do a lot of my healthy shopping online. From toothpaste, shampoo, and soaps to diapers and wipes. I began saving 20% on my purchases and received free shipping when I subscribed to Amazon Mom and chose my "subscribe and save items." Most of the products that I recommend in my book and blog are available on Amazon and qualify for the 20% discount. This is a great opportunity for you to start saving money and trips to the store. I downloaded the app on my phone and saved the credit card information, so it is very easy to make any purchases. I found it to be very helpful in checking off items from my shopping list.

Buying natural oils and products that have multiple uses is another great way to maximize your budget. Shea butter can be used as a very effective eye cream, but also doubles as a diaper rash cream and sunscreen. Tea tree oil can be used as a treatment against acne and black heads, for humidifiers, and chest rubs. Dr. Bronner's soap can be used for face, body, and washing dishes. You can dilute it in different amounts of water for different uses. Apple cider vinegar and baking soda can be used for hair treatments and for cleaning mixes. Coconut oil, traditionally used for cooking, is a very effective moisturizer and treatment for things like mosquito bites or rashes. It is also an antifungal and a great base for making your own deodorant or even adding it to smoothies to boost their nutritional value.

Action Step: Go through your beauty routine and evaluate if you need to make any changes.

Products I should stop using: _____

_____

Products I should buy: _____

_____

My new beauty routine is: _____

_____

Part Two: Bonding with Your Baby

My youngest daughter barely fits on my lap anymore, but it seems like I felt her flutters in my womb just yesterday. I hope you are enjoying every moment you have with your baby during pregnancy. You will never be more together than you are right now. Time flies, my friends. And once these days are gone, well, they're gone.

Today is a great day to start being intentional about bonding with your baby if you haven't done so already. Pregnancy is the prime time to begin establishing a mother-baby bond. I started bonding with Bella and Mila the moment I found out I was pregnant. I would tell them how much I loved them and how excited I was to meet them. I also talked to them about activities that we were going to do. For example, before working out, I would say, "Okay, get ready for some bouncing because we are going to exercise." Or I would tell them that we were about to reach our destination if we were stuck in traffic. My husband, JC, also spoke loving words to them during this time.

I remember singing to them different soothing songs, particularly in the evening before going to bed. I don't have an artistic voice, but I sang from the heart and I felt happy while I did it. I had a feeling they felt good too.

Lastly, I created an email account for each of my daughters during both of my pregnancies as soon as we decided on a name. Writing them emails became one of my favorite things to do during pregnancy. I had a pregnancy journal, but I found that emailing was much easier because I could do it from my phone whenever I felt like it, wherever I was. I emailed them pregnancy and baby shower pictures, notes on their development, and poured my heart out with loving words. Today, I continue to send them photos and stories about the cute things they do. I never cease to write to them about how much we love them and how beautiful, good, and intelligent they are. My desire is that they will treasure all those emails when they are older and have a tangible recollection of how much we have always loved each other.

Doing these things while your baby is still in your womb will help you establish your mom-baby bond—a bond that is the foundation of your future relationship. I wanted to share these practices with you so that you could do them too! Perhaps they will inspire you to come up with your own. Whatever you choose to do, do it with love, and your baby will love it too.

> **Action Step:** Think about ways you will establish your mom-baby bond during pregnancy.

Part Three: Changes By Trimester

Each pregnancy is unique. Symptoms vary by person and even different pregnancies may be different for the same woman. **Table 8.2** is meant to guide you throughout your trimesters so that you know you are not alone and have a better understanding of what your body and baby are going through.[8]

Track your baby's growth without ultrasounds and dopplers. Your practitioner may want to use ultrasound scans or a doppler to track your baby's development during prenatal visits. The medical community has regarded ultrasound scans and dopplers safe, but the FDA has issued a warning about their overuse. "[T]he radiation associated with [ultrasound imaging and heartbeat monitors] can produce effects on the body," says Robert Phillips, Ph.D., a physicist with FDA's Center for Devices and Radiological Health (CDRH). "When ultrasound enters the body, it heats the tissues slightly. In some cases, it can also produce small pockets of gas in body fluids or tissues."[9] Research regarding the safety of ultrasounds have found that their effect ranges from changing the movement and migration of cells and neurons to damaging the cells themselves.[10]

TABLE 8.2 YOUR BODY AND BABY BY TRIMESTER

	First (Week 1-12)	Second (Week 13-28)	Third (Week 29-40+)
Symptoms	You may have headaches, mood swings, and extreme tiredness. You may have to urinate frequently and get an upset stomach, heartburn, vomiting, or constipation. You may gain or lose weight, crave some foods, and dislike others.	Nausea and fatigue begin to fade for most women. You may experience body aches, such as back, abdomen, groin, or thigh pain as your baby grows. You may have some swelling and begin to see stretch marks on your abdomen, breasts, thighs, or buttocks. Inform your practitioner if you feel numbness, tingling, or itchiness to determine if it is something more serious.	Breathing difficulty and very frequent urination due to the baby getting bigger and increasing pressure on your lungs and bladder. Hemorrhoids due to pressure. (Blue Poppy Herbs and Witch Hazel are good remedies.) Trouble sleeping. Braxton-Hicks (irregular contractions). Thinning and softening of your cervix or effacing.
Your Breasts	Your breasts may be tender or swollen.	Darkening of the skin around your nipples.	Increased tenderness and leaking of a watery pre-milk called colostrum.
Your Belly	May not show yet if this is your first pregnancy. Some women don't buckle their seat belts during pregnancy in fear that it will hurt the baby in the event of an accident. The amniotic fluid in your womb is protection for your baby. It acts as a shock absorber. You should wear your seat belt so that the lap portion fits under your belly across your hips. You and your baby will be safer this way.	It will become more evident. You will notice a dark line running down your belly, called the linea nigra. This coloration is caused by the increase in pregnancy hormones. See Chapter 5 for help finding a comfortable sleeping position.	The linea nigra may darken and your belly button may stick out.
Your Baby	At first your baby is just an embryo consisting of two layers of cells from which all organs and body parts will develop. He or she will soon be about the size of a kidney bean and constantly moving, although you won't feel him or her. His or her heart is beating quickly and the intestines are forming. Earlobes, eyelids, mouth, and nose are also taking shape.[11] Your baby and all of the organs will be formed by the end of the first trimester.	In the beginning of the second trimester, your baby is about 3 1/2 inches long and weighs about 1 1/2 ounces. His or her unique fingerprints are in place. As the weeks go by, his or her skeleton starts to harden from rubbery cartilage to bone and your baby can now hear. You're likely to feel your baby.[12]	When you enter your third trimester, your baby weighs about 2 1/4 pounds. He or she can blink and has lashes. The baby's wrinkled skin is starting to smooth out as baby fat builds. Fingernails, toenails, and hair grow. Billions of neurons are forming. The average baby is over 19 inches long and almost 7 pounds at full term.[13]

Your baby's cells are rapidly working together to form the organs during your first trimester of pregnancy. This is a critical stage in your baby's development. The sound waves transmitted by the ultrasound shake the cells to result in the image. This shake can affect the formation process. Bone heats up more than tissue. So, the negative heat effects of the scans and the risk of damage to the baby's brain increase while the bones are forming during the second and third trimesters due to the high heat.

Remember that there was a time when doctors used X-rays on pregnant women. They later found that the radiation was harmful to the babies. Ultrasounds are a relatively new technology. My husband and I weren't aware of the effects of ultrasounds from the very beginning of our first pregnancy, but we decided to only do the anatomy ultrasound going forward as soon as our doctor gave us several clinical research papers on the risks. We wanted to know the sex of our baby and make sure that all of her organs were okay. However, we preferred to avoid the risk from all other ultrasounds that were not medically necessary and we would typically do just for fun or to get a new picture of the baby.

Instead of ultrasounds and dopplers, I recommend using a fetoscope, which is like a regular stethoscope that a doctor uses to hear your heartbeat but for the womb. This conventional device doesn't pose any risk to your baby, but is very effective. I was able to listen to my baby's heartbeat through this device during each of my visits.

Lastly, there is now a new blood test that allows you to learn the sex of your baby without an ultrasound. I would have also opted for this test if it was available during my pregnancies.

Action Step: Ask your health practitioner to limit the use of ultrasound to just the anatomy ultrasound and to use the fetoscope during prenatal visits.

Part Four: Let's Talk About Sex

Your sex life doesn't have to take a toll during pregnancy. In fact, most pregnant women and their husbands agree that sex is great during pregnancy. Sex is good for you and your baby. Your body releases oxytocin, the love hormone, and a happier mom makes a happy baby. You can continue to make love throughout all of your trimesters unless your practitioner indicates otherwise. "The amniotic sac and the strong muscles of the uterus protect your baby, and the mucus plug seals the cervix to help guard against infection."[14] You may need to modify positions to accommodate your growing belly, but other than that, it's "play time" as usual. Traditional positions such as man or woman on top, spooning, or rear entry are okay. But NO blowing air into your vagina. The burst of air might block a blood vessel and be life threatening for you and the baby.

During your first trimester, your sex drive may increase due to increased blood flow and hormonal changes. Some other women experience nausea and fatigue, and this may diminish their sex drive. During this trimester, it is rare you need to abstain from having sex.

Most women find the second trimester of pregnancy easier than the first, so that increases sex drive. "The vagina is more lubricated and the clitoris and vagina are more engorged. Many women will become orgasmic or multi-orgasmic for the first time during pregnancy because of this added engorgement."[15]

In your third trimester, your baby will move lower in your abdomen or "drop," so traditional positions may cause pain or spotting during or after sex. A common concern is that sex will start labor. This is unlikely to happen if your cervix is not ripe, so don't worry about preterm labor.[16]

Cuddling, spending time together, and taking turns doing something you each enjoy will help in your relationship, especially during times of less sex. You will be going through many physical changes at this stage, but help your husband understand that there are other unseen changes taking place too. Be patient with him and ask him to be patient with you too. (Share **Table 8.2** with your husband, along with JC's Epilogue on the father's role in a healthy pregnancy to help him in this process.)

Enjoy sex during pregnancy! After you deliver, there is about a six-week waiting period to have intercourse again. "A small number of couples have sex within the first month after the birth, but about half wait until at least six weeks, as do most women who have had a tear or episiotomy."[17] Make sure your husband is aware of this

during pregnancy so it does not catch him by surprise. Discussing any expectations beforehand will make this period easier.

The first six weeks include busy days (and nights) of changing diapers, breastfeeding, and adjusting to your baby's needs. Sex may not be on your mind during this time. You may feel that you barely have energy to stay up and spend time with your husband. But being intimate during this time can help you and your spouse feel connected when everything else seems to be revolving around the baby. It may even make you feel more attractive and repel the baby blues. Making out and caressing each other, a foot massage, or fellatio for dad are some alternatives to intercourse.

Many times a little bit of effort in bed will make a huge difference in the day-to-day. Intimacy will foster closeness during a time that tends to be difficult for marriage. As moms, we go above and beyond to care for our children. Let's do the same for our marriage.

Action Step: Plan a relaxing date with your husband where you guys can talk about your changes and how you both feel. Share the Epilogue at the end of the book (written by my husband), and then talk about sex. It's a win-win if you actually have some after.

We will have our romantic date on: _____

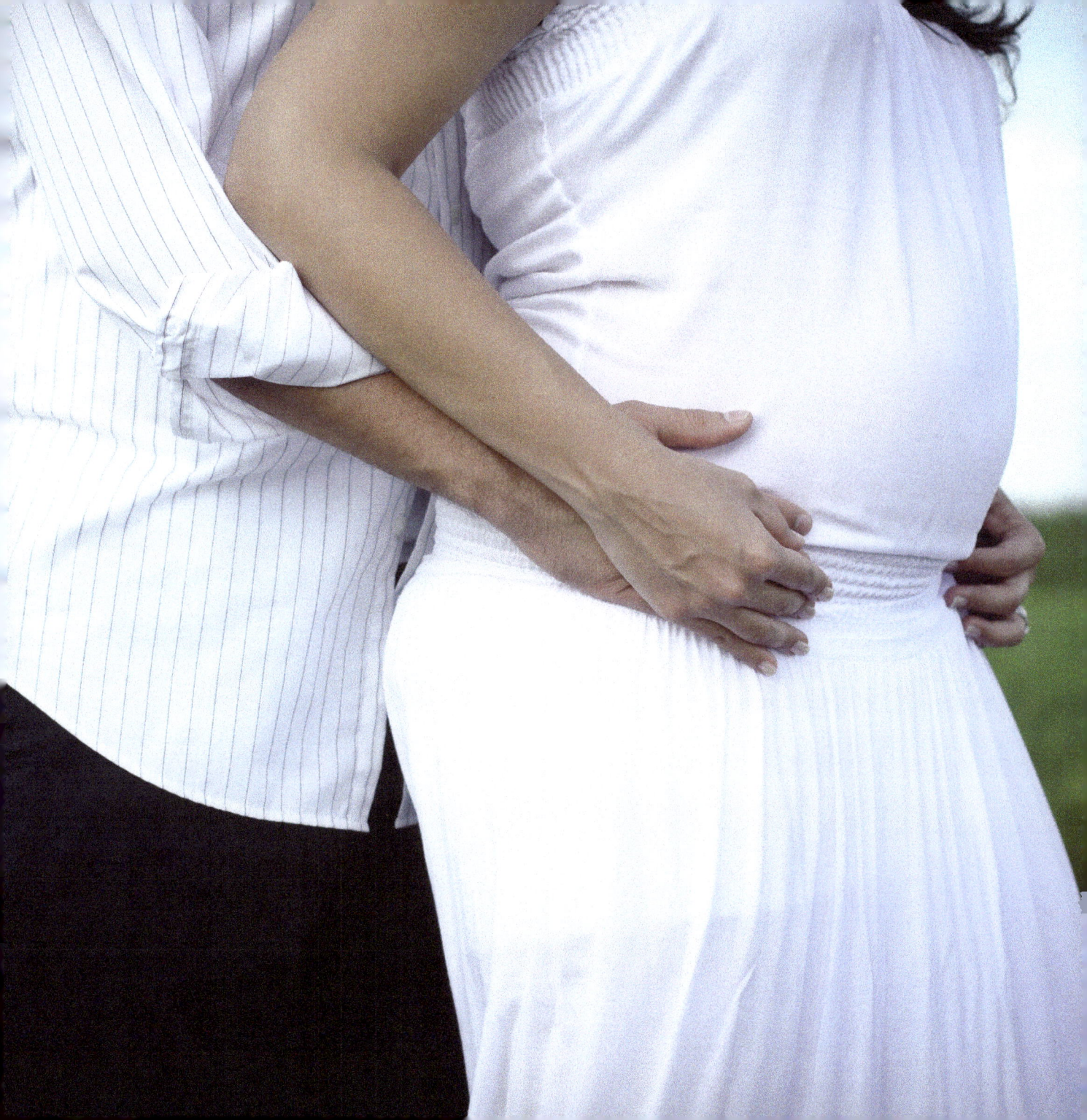

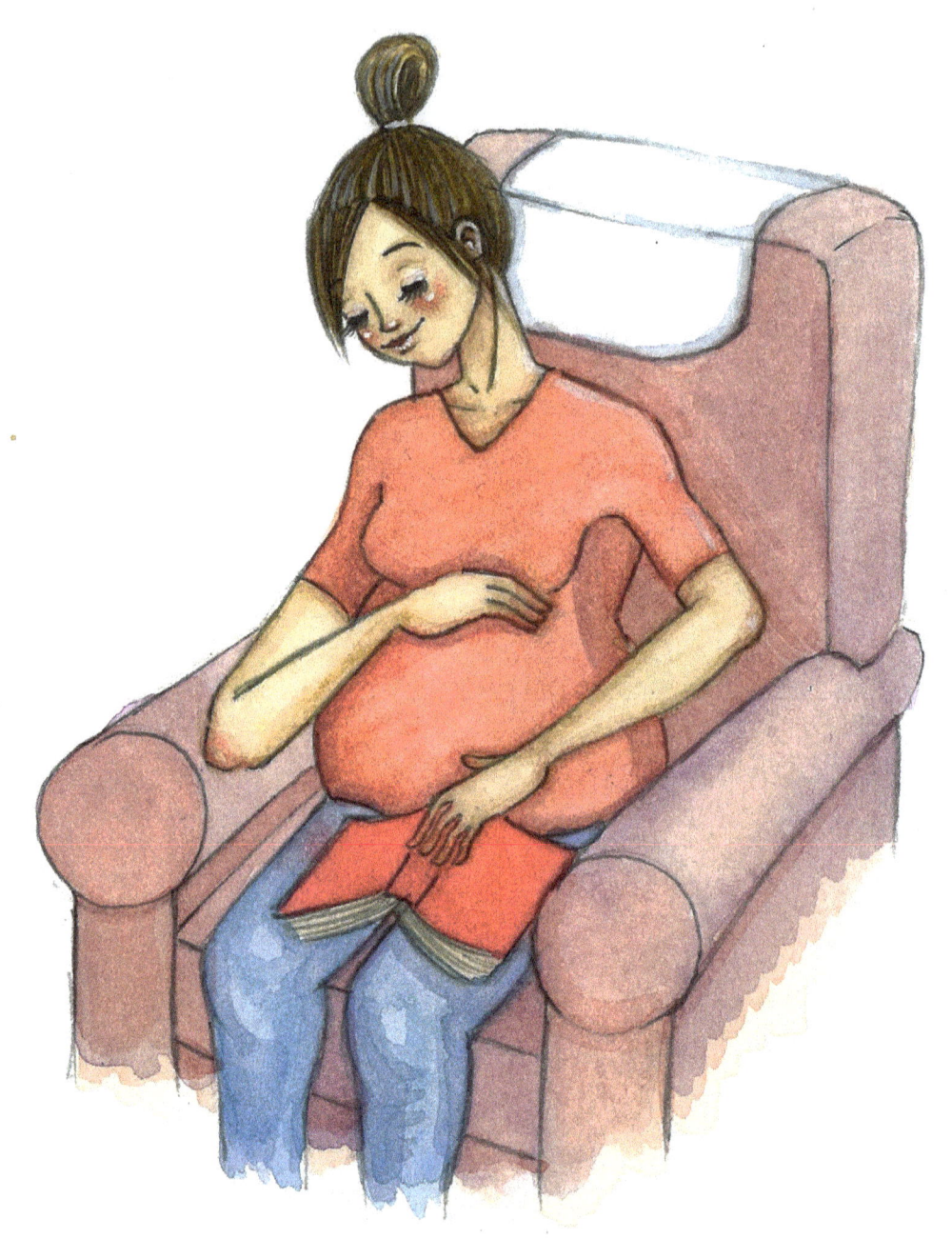

CHAPTER 9

Winning the War Against Stress

By now you know I have four kids: Abi (21), John (19), Bella (3), and Mila (1). As a young mom, I get all kinds of responses when I share about my four kids. They range from "wow, you look really young to have four kids" to "wow, you must have started very young." All of these reactions bring a smile to my face.

Chapter 13 tells the story of how my husband and I decided to adopt our older kids while we were still so young. This chapter discusses some of the tough times that we experienced when raising Abi and John during those tough teenage years and while I was pregnant with Bella and Mila. I have their permission to share these stories with you. They are very personal to us, but we hope they are beneficial to you.

Stress During my Pregnancy with Bella

I was just about to enter my third trimester with Bella. I was doing everything that I shared with you in this book so far. I was in good health and felt great. And then one Sunday I lived one of the toughest days of my life.

The day started well. I woke up, got ready, and went to church. I received tons of compliments on my belly as I walked into the service. The service was beautiful. The message the pastor shared was awesome, like usual, and I felt wonderful.

But things took a turn as I was leaving. I bumped into one of Abi's best friends who had returned home from college for summer break. She was part of the group of young girls that I led as part of our youth ministry. I loved her dearly because of how amazing she was. She was smart, witty, and charming. She was also special to me because she reminded me of my kids in a way. Her mom passed away when she was very young, and her father was incarcerated. She was a very independent girl, but in my eyes, she was in need of motherly love. This is why I had embraced her as part of our family and offered her to come live with us at one point.

I looked into her eyes and I knew that something was wrong. Abi had shared some of her friend's struggles with me, and I confirmed them when I saw her. I confronted her, encouraged her, and then offered to help her. She didn't think she needed my help, but she did feel the need to make me aware of other things regarding my own kids. She asked if we could go to my car and talk, so we did.

It was a hot summer day and I remember having the air conditioner on max. I was in the driver's seat and she was in the passenger's seat. I turned to her and prompted her to talk. She then began to unleash all of the secrets she knew about my kids. I think she shared all the mistakes Abi and John had made that she was aware of. There were so many. My heart raced faster and faster as she shared every detail. I felt like my heart was shattered by the time she was done. I was angry and sad. Disappointed. I could not wait to confront them, but not without telling JC first.

We finally confronted them in the family room of our house. It was bad. Tough. Nobody said parenting was easy. JC reminded me to calm down. I hadn't thought about the baby and the effects that this stress could have on her. I decided to take a bath and try to relax after that wake-up call. I decided to pray while taking a bath. I asked God to give me peace—to help me through it. I started doing some mental exercises that I will share with you later in this chapter, and I immediately felt a calming effect.

Looking back at that day, it was probably one of the most stressful days of my life. My faith in God really pulled me through, and so did my loving husband. Bella was born a couple of months later, and Abi and John were part of the birth. They saw their little sister be born in their

94 THE SECRETS TO A HEALTHY PREGNANCY

home. And the past was the past. We came out of that experience stronger than before and with more love toward each other.

I wish I could say that was it, but a lot more has happened since. We've lived through many difficult stages with our kids through the years. Some were better than others, but all were worth the hard work.

Stress During my Pregnancy with Mila

I also experienced high stress during Mila's pregnancy. The week I found out I was pregnant with Mila, I also found out that I was about to lose my job and $30,000 of owed commission. Not long after, I actually lost my job.

The night before I found out I was pregnant with Mila, John came home after his curfew, and JC confiscated his cell phone as a result. Throughout that night and the following day, JC learned that Abi and John were back to the life they were living while I was pregnant with Bella. But this time was even worse than before. JC shared what was happening, and although I was very upset, I learned not to let the external uncontrollable circumstances affect my baby. I waited hours to tell JC that I was pregnant and couldn't wait anymore. So, I brought the pregnancy test and told him I was pregnant. He was very happy.

John kept rebelling throughout the next six months of my pregnancy with Mila. He was coming home late, cutting school, failing all his classes, and getting into lots of trouble. We gave him chance after chance and even went to counseling, but he wouldn't improve. JC and I listened to podcasts on parenting and sought advice from our best friends and church. One day we realized that we needed to be clear with him. We could not allow his lifestyle in our home. So we sat with him and told him he had three more strikes, and after that, if he persisted in his ways, we would understand that he did not want to comply with the house rules and was therefore choosing to move out.

I was eight months pregnant with Mila the day that John decided to leave the house. That was really tough for all of us, but I felt peace. We knew there was nothing else we could do to help him. We had to let him go. Our parents, my church pastors, and friends were great support. They encouraged me to think about Mila and my health during my pregnancy. They all prayed for us at church on the Sunday after John left.

I continued eating healthy, exercising, and doing my chiropractic and naturopathic care. I felt peace even in the midst of all the chaos. John came home three weeks later. We forgave him and embraced him. That's what parenting is all about—being there for your kids when they need you. Sometimes they don't even realize

that they need you and want to do things their way. You can set up rules and enforce them. You can implement consequences, but you cannot change their heart. Only God can do that.

I pray for our kids every day—from the smallest to the oldest. I pray for their faith and their future. Having children comes with so much responsibility, worries, and sleepless nights. But it is definitely worth it. The joy, the happy moments, and the rewarding feeling that you get when you see them learn and grow make it all worth it.

I wanted to share these stories with you so you would know that my pregnancies were not just a breeze or a walk in the park. I experienced a lot of stress in the midst of them, but I pulled through. I didn't let stress get a hold of me. Instead, I managed it, and my baby and I remained healthy.

Why Stress is Bad

You may have heard there is good stress and bad stress. Both of them release the stress hormone cortisol. The difference lies in that one has an outlet that brings back balance and the other doesn't. Eustress, the good stress, creates a "seize-the-day" heightened state of arousal, which is invigorating and often linked with a tangible goal. This is the stress that you get from exercising or riding a roller coaster. After the task is completed, cortisol levels return to normal. Distress, the bad stress, doesn't provide an outlet for the cortisol and causes the fight-or-flight mechanism to backfire.[1] This build-up in the blood creates distress on your mind and body.

Scientists have known for years that elevated cortisol levels interfere with learning and memory; lower immune function and bone density; and increase weight gain, blood pressure, cholesterol, and heart disease. Chronic stress and elevated cortisol levels also increase risk for depression, mental illness, and lower life expectancy.[2]

Stress also lowers your immune system. Just the fact that you are pregnant makes you prone to infections, colds, and flus. Remember that your immune system is lowered slightly during pregnancy in order to stop your body from rejecting your baby who is competing with you for resources. The result is an even weaker you when you add stress to this equation.

Chronic stress, or too much of the bad stress, can result in sleep deprivation, headaches, loss of appetite, or the opposite—a tendency to overeat—all of which can be harmful to you and your developing baby.

My naturopath, Dr. Gisela Hernandez, takes the emotional state of the pregnant woman into ac-

count when suggesting treatment options. She explained to me that an altered emotional state could affect the nervous system and the healing process and that stress can cause someone to become sick or affect an existing illness. The immune system has a fundamental role in the process of healing. Studies reveal that people who are under chronic stress have low white blood cell counts and their immune systems are more vulnerable.[3]

How Stress Affects Your Baby

High stress levels can cause high blood pressure, which increases your chance of having preterm labor or a low-birth-weight baby.[4] Research also reveals that cortisol appears to cross the placenta and may affect your baby and disturb ongoing developmental processes.[5] Researchers, led by Professor Vivette Glover in London, examined the relationship between the stress hormones in the mother's blood and stress hormones present in the amniotic fluid around the baby in the womb. They studied 267 women, taking a blood sample from the mother and a sample from the amniotic fluid surrounding the baby.

"Early in the second trimester, your baby starts to swallow the [amniotic] fluid, pass it through his kidneys, and excrete it as urine, which he then swallows again, recycling the full volume of amniotic fluid every few hours."[6] At this stage, your baby is, in essence, producing the amniotic fluid, so the fluid's composition reflects your baby's exposure to various substances, including hormones. The researchers measured the levels of cortisol present in both samples at gestational age of 17 weeks or greater. They found that the higher the cortisol levels in the mother's blood, the greater was the level of cortisol in the amniotic fluid.[7]

Professor Glover has studied more than 7,000 women. She has showed how stress and anxiety during pregnancy can affect an unborn baby's mental and emotional development.[8] In one of her studies *Children of the 1990s*, she found that women who were anxious in the last trimester of pregnancy had children with more behavioral problems. Those who had boys were twice as likely to have a child with hyperactivity and ADHD by age four.[9]

Even after considering family history of ADHD and other environmental factors, studies link maternal stress during pregnancy with the development of ADHD.[10] Other studies reveal that "children with ADHD whose mothers underwent moderate and severe stress during pregnancy tend to develop more severe symptoms than children with ADHD whose mothers were not exposed to prenatal stress."[11] Lastly, research even ties depression during pregnancy to having a baby that is prone to being unhappy from birth on.[12]

Stress Remedies

It's normal to feel some stress during pregnancy. Your body is going through many changes and your moods change as your hormones change. You begin worrying about a new life forming inside of you. You become very protective and even a little paranoid. However, it is important to create outlets for that stress. From communicating your anxieties to exercising, there are tools within your reach that will help ensure your healthy pregnancy goes on.

Here are some tools that helped me fight stress during pregnancy. These are my antidotes to cortisol. Just like greater messes require more paper towels, the more stress you face, the more I advise you to use these antidotes. I created an acronym to help you fight stress: REACT.

"R" is for Rest. Research shows that napping regularly may reduce stress and even decrease your risk of heart disease.[13] Stress can sometimes affect your evening sleep; so napping may complement your evening sleep so that you have enough rest to function throughout the day. Chapter 5 has plenty of information on the healthy effects of naps.

"E" is for Exercise. Virtually any form of exercise, from aerobics to walking, can act as a stress reliever. Exercise is a great way to reduce stress levels, and your baby will enjoy the serotonin and endorphins that your body produces. Regular exercise can increase self-confidence and lower the symptoms associated with anxiety. Exercise can also improve your sleep, which is often affected during pregnancy.

"A" is for Alternative Medicine. Chiropractic, acupuncture, and naturopathic care have methods of reducing stress levels. I am a fan of alternative medicine because I found it is more focused on addressing the cause and not the symptoms. Many healthcare plans cover alternative medicine treatments. I also found that getting adjusted by a chiropractor during pregnancy helped me feel better and more relaxed right away.

"C" is for Communicate. When struggling with a stressful situation, it may be helpful to talk with someone you can trust. Venting to your spouse or friend can be very therapeutic. If you are feeling stress about pregnancy or motherhood it is important you let your midwife or doctor know. They have a lot of helpful information to ease your concerns. My midwife always had the right words to say whenever I had doubts about anything. I'm so glad I got to benefit from her wise counsel. All I had to do was open up.

"T" is for Take Action or Let it Go. Assess whether the situation requires an action from your part. There are some things you can solve with actions. There are others you can put on hold. There are others you can't do anything about. Either way, some degree of action is required from you from the action of fixing the issue to the action of letting go. Stressing or worrying about them isn't going to help. As a matter a fact, it's just going to hurt you and your baby. If your assessment reveals there is an action required from your part, then go for it. But if there is nothing you can do to aid in the situation, then let it go.

How My Faith Helps Me Let Go

Dr. Walter Calvert conducted a study of the things we worry about. He found that we spend 92% of our emotional energies on things that won't happen or things we can't change.[14]

My friend Samantha L. called me while I was at Starbucks writing this very chapter. She was 32 weeks pregnant and in the middle of selling her house and moving into a new home. She had many tasks to complete. As she approached her due date, her stress levels increased because her home was not yet ready, and she was planning a home birth. I listened to her realizing she had been crying and offered to pray for her. Afterwards, I shared with her this little tip that I have as part of my "letting go" mechanism. It's called "Count to 10 and let it go."

The first thing I do is pray about my problem. Prayer was, and still is, vital to me during periods of high stress. I ask God to take my anxiety and direct me in any way I need to be directed. I pray for His peace. This is not a magic formula but I have included it to help you come up with your own.

> *Dear God,*
>
> *Thank you for being here for me. I believe you listen to my prayers and have the power to help me. I don't want to be anxious anymore. I give you my problem. Please help me take care of it. I trust you.*
>
> *In Jesus' name, Amen.*

Take a very deep breath after praying and picture your anxieties evaporating. This doesn't mean they will magically go away, but it helps release the stress. In your mind, begin counting to 10 while you continue taking slow deep breaths. The slower you go, the better. It helps me to raise my hands as if I am surrendering and letting God take it all. Imagine that the problem is dissolving with each deep breath you take. The goal is to allow your mind to let go of the problem once you reach 10.

This Bible verse encourages us to do this so that we can have peace: "Do not be anxious about anything, but in every situation, by prayer and petition, with thanksgiving, present your requests to God. And the peace of God, which transcends all understanding, will guard your hearts and your minds in Christ Jesus." (Philippians 4:6-7.)

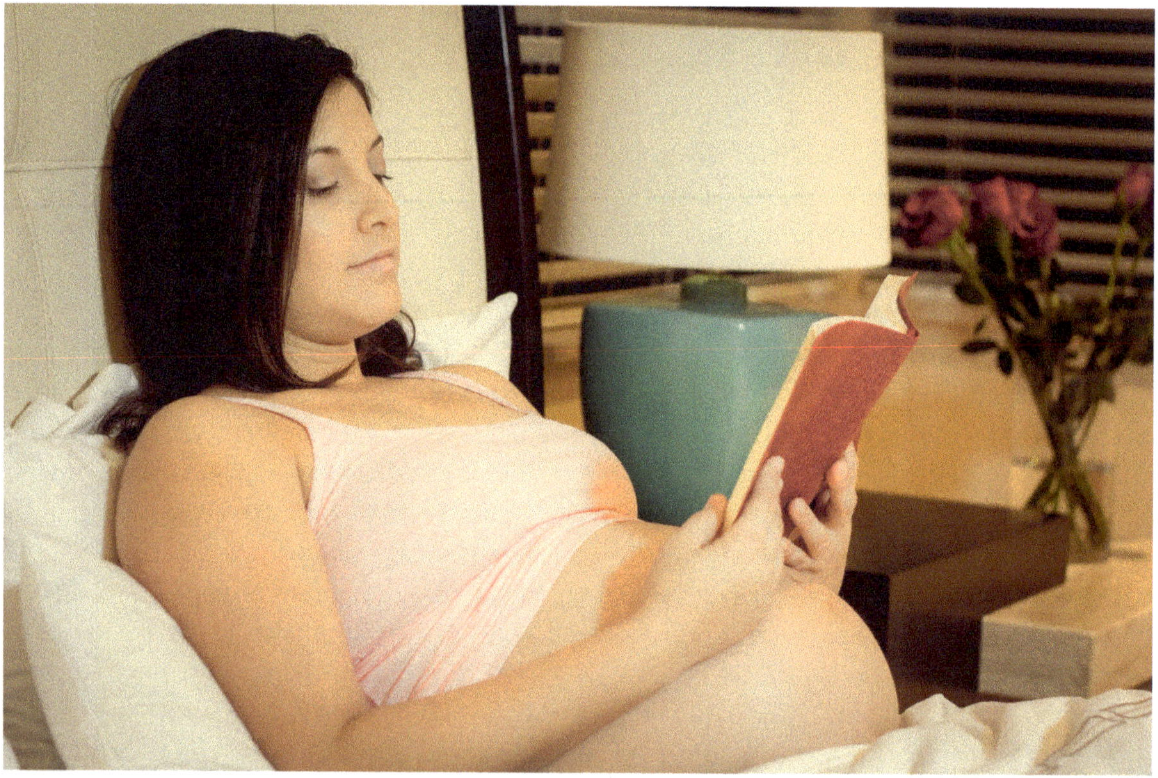

Reliving the memories in this chapter has been challenging. I hope it helped you and I connect as humans in this experience of life where nothing is perfect—even during pregnancy. Even though it would be great if the world realized we were pregnant and somehow gave us a pass to get out of every stressful situation, it doesn't work that way. But that's okay. You can surpass your tough moments, just like I surpassed mine. Then, your story will encourage someone else, and so on. Every difficult situation is an opportunity. Even though they may hurt, these experiences make us stronger and give us the opportunity to help one another. Knowing my difficulties aren't just about me and that I have the power to use them to bless another person encourages me during those tough times. You have that power too. Use it.

Samantha L. went into labor eight weeks after our phone conversation. I was with her during the last stages of her first natural childbirth. Seeing her labor in her clean, organized, and lovely new home filled me with joy. The stress of moving was long gone. She focused on her breathing and, like a lioness, delivered a healthy baby boy in her big bathtub.

Before you know it you will be holding your baby in your arms and may even find yourself missing pregnancy—a time when you and your baby were more connected than ever. So don't let stress rob you of this precious time of bonding with your baby in your womb! Instead, enjoy your pregnancy!

Action Step: Go through the R.E.A.C.T. acronym and see what areas you can be better at. Then, do something about it.

R _____

E _____

A _____

C _____

T _____

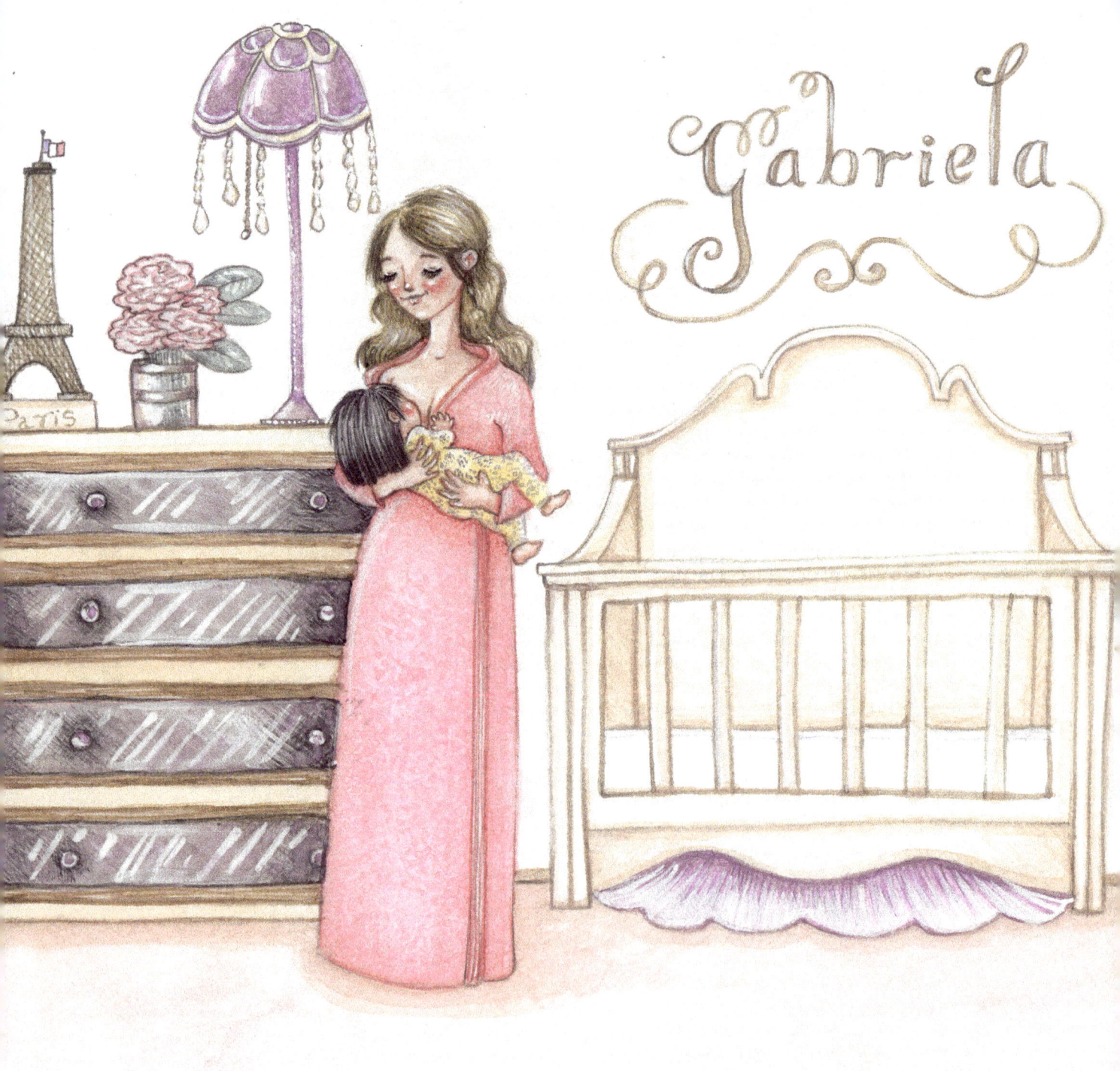

CHAPTER 10

Preparing to Breastfeed Successfully

I really wanted to breastfeed. I thought it was an amazing and beautiful thing. My mom nursed me as an infant, and one of my best friends, Samantha C., was currently breastfeeding and was very passionate about it. Everything I read in preparation for Bella's birth taught me that it was the healthiest way to go.

I wanted to breastfeed so badly that one night, while I was still pregnant with Bella, I dreamt that I was nursing her as a newborn while walking down an aisle at the supermarket. My friend Tanya saw how badly I wanted to breastfeed, so she recommended I visit a lactation consultant before giving birth. This would ensure we were well informed and ready before we even began the process.

I met with the lactation consultant when I was about 35 weeks pregnant. She asked me to bring the persons who would be supporting me after birth, so I brought my husband and my mom. The lactation consultant shared with us very helpful information about breastfeeding and showed us a few educational videos. This is when I learned about the breast crawl.

Learning about the breast crawl was great. I did it with both Bella and Mila just minutes after they were born. The breast crawl consists of placing your baby on you while you are at a semi-reclined position and letting him or her breastfeed on their own. Your baby will be able to smell the milk and literally crawl to your breast and begin nursing. It is a beautiful sight.

Before the session was over, she also examined my breasts. She said the fact that my veins were visible through my skin was a good sign because it indicated increased blood flow to the breasts. The fact that my bra size increased a cup size during pregnancy was another good sign. She did point out that there was a lot of space between my breasts, which can sometimes be a sign of underdeveloped breast tissue. This could lead to difficulty producing enough milk. Although she was very positive and encouraging, she recommended that I take Goat's Rue by Mother Love as a preventive measure. Goat's Rue is an herb that helps build mammary tissue, and is safe to take during pregnancy.

My naturopath also recommended that I eat sesame seeds, which are believed to help with milk production. Unfortunately, I didn't do so. I didn't really worry about breastfeeding apart from the visit I had with the lactation consultant. I didn't even take the Goat's Rue; the associate at a small health food store sold me another Mother Love product by mistake due to similar packaging.

I started breastfeeding immediately after Bella was born. She latched on right away when we were still in the bathtub where she was born. I made sure to include breastfeeding as part of my birth plan. Breastfeeding was smooth until day two. Bella was so excited when my milk transitioned from colostrum to milk that she nursed enthusiastically for a long time.[1] A friend came to visit me, and I was distracted talking to her. I didn't notice the lapse of time until she left. Bella had nursed herself to sleep, but I left her sucking for two hours afterwards. I didn't notice at the moment, but the next day my nipples were raw. Here are the most important lessons I learned from this and other experiences while nursing Bella and Mila.

Moderate the Nursing Times to Prevent Raw Nipples

I never thought this would happen to me, but it is very common. Many lactation consultants say that a good latch should not cause raw nipples. However, your nipples may get very sore, even with a good latch. I believe Bella had a good latch, and my nipples still cracked because of prolonged nursing early on. Once you see your baby has finished drinking and is now asleep, carefully unlatch him or her. The way to do it is by sticking your index finger in your baby's mouth and opening it so you can undo the latch. Then, you can separate your breast from the mouth. To prevent hurting yourself, do not pull before undoing the latch.

I endured the raw nipples stage by applying coconut oil frequently. I also applied some of my own breast milk. I would squirt a little on my finger and rub it. Some recommend using Lanolin in extreme cases like mine, but I wanted to stay as natural as possible.

Breastfeeding became easier when my nipples healed and I got used to nursing Bella many times throughout the day. But I felt like a giant pacifier. My friend Tanya came to visit me and really encouraged me. She told me that this stage doesn't last very long and that it would get better. And it did.

Enjoy Nursing Your Infant

I expected breastfeeding to be awesome all the time and never expected to feel tired of it. At first, I felt like I couldn't do anything because I was always sitting down nursing. But that stage was soon over, and I missed it afterwards. I was

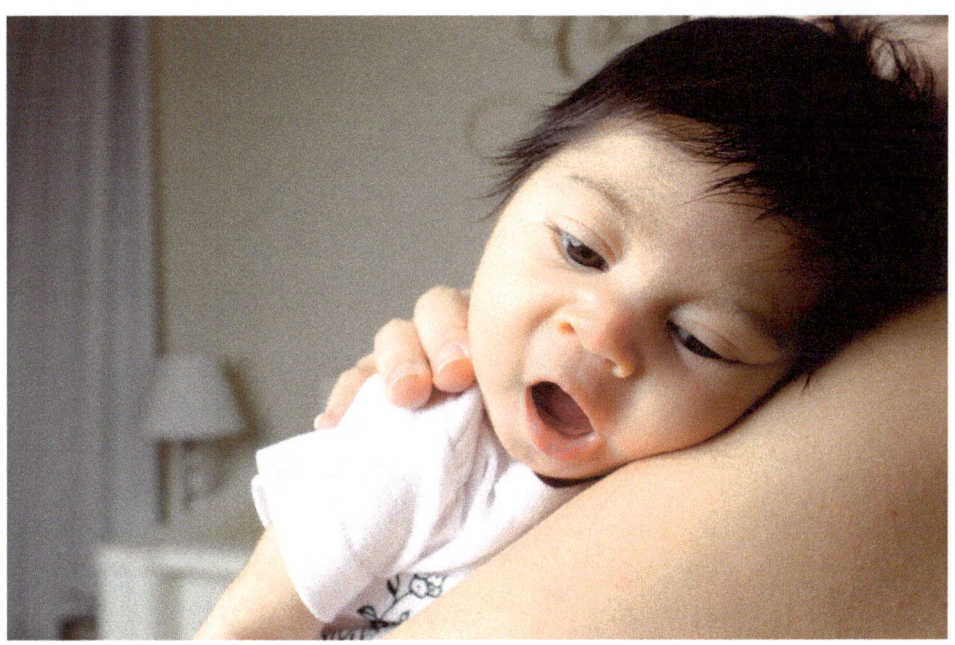

BELLA 2 MONTHS

running around trying to keep up with my crawling baby after just a few months. God knows what is best for your baby. This time of nursing is the time for you and your baby to get to know each other. To bond. To stare into each other's eyes. Smell your baby. Kiss your baby. Caress your baby's soft skin. They grow so fast. Every parent knows that this stage flies by. You will have a toddler, and you will be running around trying to keep him or her out of trouble before you know it!

Keep Track of Your Baby's Weight

International Board Certified lactation consultant, Anne Smith, says, "One of the biggest concerns all new moms have is whether or not their baby is gaining enough weight, especially when they are breastfeeding."[2]

Bella was three weeks old when I finally felt confident breastfeeding. I also felt more confident driving around with her by this time, so I accepted an invitation to attend a breastfeeding support group. I went to the group and felt comforted by seeing all the other mothers breastfeeding. The lactation consultants had a scale to weigh the babies and see if they were gaining enough weight. They were concerned when they weighed Bella. They thought she wasn't drinking enough milk because she was at her same birth weight.

Here is something very important for you to know about birth weight: a five to seven percent weight loss during the first three to four days after birth is normal. A ten percent weight loss is sometimes considered normal, but this amount of weight loss is a sign that you need to evaluate the breastfeeding. It's a good idea to have a routine weight check at five days because the baby should be gaining rather than losing weight by then. By doing so, you can catch and remedy any developing problems early on. Always calculate weight gain from the lowest point instead of doing it from the baby's birth weight. Your baby should reach his or her birth weight by day ten to fourteen.[3]

In addition, make sure the baby is weighed on the same scale and preferably naked each time to get an accurate picture of the weight gain. Different scales can give very different readings. You can ask your midwife or pediatrician to do this. The practitioner should use the 2006 WHO standards because older ones include less breastfed children that tend to grow faster and be heavier. My mistake was not weighing Bella on the second week. If I had, I would have noticed something was off and began an improvement plan sooner.

Be Careful with the Tongue-Tie Myth

The lactation consultants proceeded to evaluate Bella's latch and determined it was fine. Then they examined her tongue to check if she may be tongue-tied. This is when the frenulum (the band of tissue that connects the bottom of the tongue to the floor of the mouth) is too short and tight, causing the movement of the tongue to be restricted. One of them said that Bella was indeed tongue-tied and that it may be hindering her from drinking enough milk. She referred me to a pediatrician that could do a frenetomy—a procedure in which the doctor clips the frenulum to loosen it and allow the tongue full range of motion. However, the pediatrician examined her and determined that Bella did not have a tongue-tie.

It has become very common to diagnose infants with tongue-tie. We must be careful with this. I believe in minimizing unnecessary interventions that may sometimes lead to other complications. My midwife and pediatrician checked Bella's tongue during her first check-up and thought it was fine, but the lactation consultant was convinced Bella was tongue-tied. Don't be afraid to ask for a second opinion. My chiropractor, Dr. Lisa, provided me with lots of articles on how tongue-tie may resolve itself independently. There are babies with tongue-ties that nurse perfectly.[4] Some tongue-ties also loosen over time on their own.[5]

You Can Supplement With Someone Else's Breast Milk

I scheduled a home visit with a lactation consultant to evaluate Bella's milk intake during a feeding. She weighed Bella before and after nursing and concluded that Bella wasn't drinking enough milk. She said it was necessary for me to supplement right away because I didn't have enough milk to fulfill Bella's needs. I was devastated, and I felt inadequate. She told me I had to supplement with formula. But I remembered learning during a prenatal class that you could supplement with someone else's breast milk.

I immediately thought of my friend, Samantha C., and called her crying. I asked her if she could help me, and she said yes. Samantha pumped milk for me for the next three weeks until my milk supply was established. This experience brought us closer together as friends. We shared a special bond. Consider using a friend that shares similar eating and nutritional habits if you plan on doing something like this. This task is a big undertaking. Samantha pumped for me and nursed her toddler. This can cause some

engorgement and clogged ducts due to increased milk supply. It can typically be resolved with more pumping, but is something to keep in mind for the person giving the milk. Pumping for a friend is a beautiful act of friendship. I am forever grateful for her love and friendship during this time. JC and I made her Bella's godmother, and I feel that they will always share that special bond.

You Can Take Steps to Increase Your Milk Supply

I worked on increasing my milk supply during the time Samantha pumped for me. The lactation consultant told me I could be part of the 1% of women who could not nurse exclusively. But I didn't let that discourage me—I was determined to make it work. It took about three weeks for my milk supply to regulate after following these steps:

Increase demand through pumping. Breastfeeding is a supply and demand relationship. Use a hospital-grade pump to get the best results. I rented a hospital pump until a friend let me borrow hers. I pumped for ten minutes after every feeding. This is not about pumping milk out, so do not be discouraged by how much comes out. Man-made pumps do not draw out breast milk like a baby. This is about letting your body know that it needs to produce more. Pumping after every breastfeeding session ensures that your breasts are empty and will also send a message to your body to produce more milk.

Take supplements. I took three tablets of fenugreek and marshmallow root with every meal. You can take these after the baby is born. For those of you who prefer supplements in liquid form, you can take More Milk Plus by Mother Love instead. The formula contains fenugreek, blessed thistle, nettle, and fennel seed. Mother Love also sells More Milk Special Blend, which has goat's rue in addition to the More Milk Plus formula. You can see results as fast as 48 hours for cases of low milk production and within two to three weeks in cases of underdeveloped mammary tissue.

Supplement with a nursing supplementer and not with bottles in order to avoid nipple confusion. Nipple confusion occurs when a baby is given a bottle or pacifier and then forgets how to nurse.[6] A nursing supplementer is a baby bottle where the nipple is cut a little bit bigger to allow a thin tube to pass through the opening. This bottle is filled with your expressed breast milk or donor breast milk. As soon as your baby latches, you sneak in the tube through the side of your baby's mouth. As the baby nurses, milk from your breast and the supplementer is drawn into his or her mouth. "A supplementer allows you to make sure your baby is getting enough nutrition while continuing to stimulate your body to produce and build up your breast milk supply."[7]

Breastfeed on demand. I didn't have a fixed breastfeeding schedule because that could lower my milk supply. This is true especially during growth spurts that happen approximately between one and three weeks, six and eight weeks, three months, six months, and nine months.[8]

Eat better. Looking back, I wasn't eating well in the beginning of Bella's life. I was so consumed with caring after a newborn that I neglected my own nutrition. I think that is why I lost weight so fast and also why I may have had those initial issues with breastfeeding.

Hire a lactation consultant. Visit a lactation consultant at around 35 weeks to prepare for breastfeeding. Some will give you a preferred rate for mom and baby consultation if you were a prenatal patient. Not all lactation consultants are the same. Ask your friends that breastfeed for recommendations.

Eat Like You are Still Pregnant—and then Eat Some More

I believe that my diet was one of the factors that may have hindered my milk production. I don't think I was having enough protein to sustain me as a vegetarian. I went back to my pre-pregnancy weight one week after having Bella. I think I was focused more on my weight and not on making sure that I was eating enough. I also think I was so busy adjusting my life to caring after a newborn, that I neglected my own nutrition.

You need more calories when you nurse than when you are pregnant. According to the AAP and Kelly Mom, you need to consume 250 extra calories per day during pregnancy and 500 extra per day when breastfeeding. Breastfeeding is very taxing on your body. I found that eating fresh farm foods during my pregnancy with Mila helped me produce more milk. I also made it a goal to eat plenty of protein-rich foods and healthy fats those first days after giving birth. Consider adding a calcium supplement to your diet. I took two tablets of Calcium with Vitamin D by Nature's Sunshine before bedtime.

I breastfed Bella exclusively until six months. I then began giving her a soft boiled egg yolk at night and slowly introduced foods based on my vegetarian adaptation of the Weston Price Diet.

In retrospect, I should have prepared better for breastfeeding. There is no doubt that breast milk is the best food for your baby. Why leave its success to chance? Don't neglect to prepare for this very important task, which impacts your baby's health in so many ways.

Breastfeeding is Harder than Labor

Many women agree that breastfeeding is more difficult than labor because it goes on much longer. We are also so caught up in preparing for the birth, that we don't have accurate expectations of how demanding and consuming breastfeeding is. Don't get me wrong, breastfeeding is amazing! It is one of the most rewarding things I have ever done in my life. I am glad I didn't give up, but it is hard.

It is no surprise that more than 70% of American women don't follow the recommendations that they should exclusively breastfeed their babies for the first six months.[9] Health care companies and government entities are encouraging women to breastfeed because they know the many benefits it brings to both moms and babies.

It helps to have a support group of breastfeeding moms. A great support group can be your closest friends who have successfully breastfed. The first weeks tend to be the hardest ones. It can take a toll on you physically, mentally, and emotionally. Having that close group of friends may be very beneficial during those difficult moments. If you have a moment of desperation, and feel like quitting, please contact a lactation consultant first. She can help with issues like the baby not latching, nipple problems, and much more. You can find a support group and a lactation consultant near you at La Leche League's website, *www.lll.org*.

There are huge barriers to successful breastfeeding—from the lack of information on its benefits to the sexualization of breasts. This last one causes embarrassment among women who breastfeed in public. It leads them to conceal breastfeeding to the point of feeling like they have to go to a bathroom or closet to breastfeed. I have experienced this pressure, and it's important we do more to support breastfeeding moms. Supporting women who breastfeed can help them better accommodate the demands of everyday life while protecting their infants' health and contributing to a healthier adult life.

The longer you breastfeed the more confident you will become. My husband and I felt comfortable breastfeeding our babies anywhere, as long as I had my cover. I tried a few ones and even made my own. My favorite is Bebe Au Lait Bebe's Nursing Cover (about $30) because of its coverage, durability, and visibility of the baby while nursing.

The Many Mutual Benefits of Breastfeeding

Table 10.1 lists some of the numerous benefits of breastfeeding and extended breastfeeding. Come back to this table whenever you are struggling with breastfeeding and take joy and pride that you are playing a vital role in your baby's health and development. You can also use this table when others ask you why you are *still* breastfeeding.

TABLE 10.1 BENEFITS OF BREASTFEEDING

	Benefit of Breastfeeding	Prolonged Breastfeeding
Baby's Health	Human milk contains nutrients, antibodies, and immune-modulating substances that are *not* present in infant formula or cow's milk.[10] They protect infants from bacteria and viruses.	It is recommend that babies be *exclusively breastfed for the first 6 months* and that breastfeeding continue for *at least* 12 months, and thereafter for as long as mutually desired.[11]
	Breastfeeding is an unequalled way of providing ideal food for the healthy growth and development of infants.[12]	As a global public health recommendation, infants should be exclusively breastfed for the first six months of life to achieve optimal growth, development and health. Thereafter, to meet their evolving nutritional requirements, infants should receive nutritionally adequate and safe complementary foods while breastfeeding continues for up to two years of age or beyond.[13]
	Breastfed children have fewer ear, respiratory, and urinary tract infections, and have diarrhea less often.	Children weaned before two years of age are at increased risk of illness.[14]
	Infants who are exclusively breastfed tend to need fewer healthcare visits, prescriptions, and hospitalizations, resulting in a lower total medical care cost compared to never-breastfed infants.	Breastfeeding toddlers between the ages of one and three have been found to have fewer illnesses, illnesses of shorter duration, and lower mortality rates[15]
	Breastfeeding lowers risk of obesity.[16]	Breast milk is easy to digest and very nutritious, and your baby decides how much and when to eat. This helps your baby develop healthy eating patterns.[17]
	Having been breastfed is associated with decreased risk of breast cancer.[18]	Some of the immune factors in breast milk increase in concentration during the second year and also during the weaning process.[19]

TABLE 10.1 CONT'D...

	Benefit of Breastfeeding	Prolonged Breastfeeding
Child's Development	Extensive research on the relationship between cognitive achievement (IQ scores, grades in school) and breastfeeding has shown the greatest gains for those children breastfed the longest.[20]	
	A couple of studies have shown a positive relationship between longer breastfeeding duration and social and physiological development (including gross motor, fine motor, receptive language, expressive language, social-emotional, self help and cognitive function.)[21]	
	Breastfeeding promotes a growing attachment between mom and baby—from hormonal activity to emotional closeness—that will continue to play an important role in your baby's development for years to come.[22]	
Mother's Health	Earlier return to pre-pregnancy weight.[23]	Studies have found a significant inverse association between duration of lactation and breast cancer risk.[24]
	Reduces risk of pre-menopausal breast cancer and osteoporosis.	Longer breastfeeding duration is further associated with reduced maternal risks of breast cancer, ovarian cancer, diabetes, hypertension, obesity, and heart attack.[25]
	Breastfeeding is an integral part of the reproductive process with important implications for the health of mothers.[26]	Extended nursing delays the return of fertility in some women by suppressing ovulation.[27]
	Reduces the risk of rheumatoid arthritis.[28]	
	Reduces the risk of cardiovascular disease.[29]	
	Breastfeeding has been shown to decrease insulin requirements in diabetic women. There is also a decreased risk of Type 2 diabetes mellitus in mothers who do not have a history of gestational diabetes.[30]	
Financial	Based on how much milk an infant consumes the first 12 months and a formula price of $0.19/ounce, you will save an average of $1,733.75 in formula powder. This calculation excludes indirect costs, such as additional nutritional needs for a nursing mother, as well as bottles and water for formula.[31]	When you are away from home, you can feed your baby without the need to spend on a snack. In other words, you always have a healthy meal on hand.

Establishing a Breastfeeding Goal

Determine how long you want to breastfeed for and establish a goal. Doing this before you start breastfeeding will be very encouraging while you are doing it, especially during the first weeks when you feel like all you do is breastfeed. I initially wanted to breastfeed for one year, but that increased to two years once I saw how my baby was healthier than others and how special our bond was.

Breastfeeding is hard and I felt like quitting many times. But I am so happy I didn't. I reminded myself of why I was doing this and thought about my goal during those moments of frustration. Think about your breastfeeding goal and write it down on **Action Item 10.2**. List all the reasons you want to breastfeed including those I may have left out.

ACTION ITEM 10.2 MY BREASTFEEDING GOAL

My goal is to nurse until my baby is _____ old, because:

You Can Breastfeed Through Pregnancy

Bella was one year old when JC and I began trying to conceive again, and I became pregnant with Mila right away. I knew that nursing Bella could help me transition into nursing Mila. I thought she would help with milk supply and any engorgement issues. It would also help with their bonding. So I decided NOT to stop nursing Bella when I found out I was pregnant with Mila. Nursing Bella to sleep for naptime and bedtime made it easier for me to get a moment of peace and quiet. Putting her to bed was easy. Nursing is a great way to get a toddler to cool down. I am also convinced that Bella helped in my success breastfeeding Mila. I did not experience sore breasts because I never stopped nursing. So, do not be afraid to continue breastfeeding. It can actually help you during pregnancy and those first months of breastfeeding your younger child.

Two is Better Than One When it Comes to Nursing

Tandem nursing is when two siblings of different ages nurse during the same period of time. This typically happens because the older baby was too young to wean and continued nursing throughout a pregnancy.[32] "Children younger than two years of age are at increased risk of illness if weaned. Breastfeeding the nursing child after delivery of the next child may help provide a smooth psychological transition for the older child."[33] Most mothers nurse each child separately. They do not have both children at their breasts at the exact same time. The oldest usually nurses only after the younger child is finished. Other breastfeeding mothers, however, actually enjoy the opportunity to nurse both children together. They claim this lessens sibling rivalry and fosters a special bond between their children.[34] It was really nice to tandem nurse for the first couple of months after Mila was born, and Bella really enjoyed it. There is a popular book called *Adventures in Tandem Nursing* that offers more insight on this topic.

Breastfeeding is an Art

Breastfeeding is natural, but it doesn't always come naturally. Many women want to breastfeed, but give up earlier than planned because of lack of knowledge, frustration, or desperation. Make sure you have all the tools you will need and prepare for that special period during your pregnancy. That way, when you stop, it's not because you felt like giving up but because you planned it accordingly. Let it be an accomplishment for yourself.

Learn as much as you can about breastfeeding. My favorite website for information on breastfeeding is *www.kellymom.com*. You can find lots of helpful information on the benefits of breastfeeding, how your diet impacts your milk, common baby problems, such as reflux, and so much more. If you end up supplementing with formula, the Weston A. Price foundation (*www.westonaprice.org*) has a great recipe to make your own using goat's milk. They also have a helpful timeline for the introduction of first foods.

Breastfeeding for any length of time is a success. Don't ever feel guilty for not breastfeeding "long enough." One day is better than nothing at all, and two days are better than one. Whatever you do, do it with love, and you will be just fine.

Action Step: Visit a lactation specialist for a prenatal consultation.

Visit will be on: _____

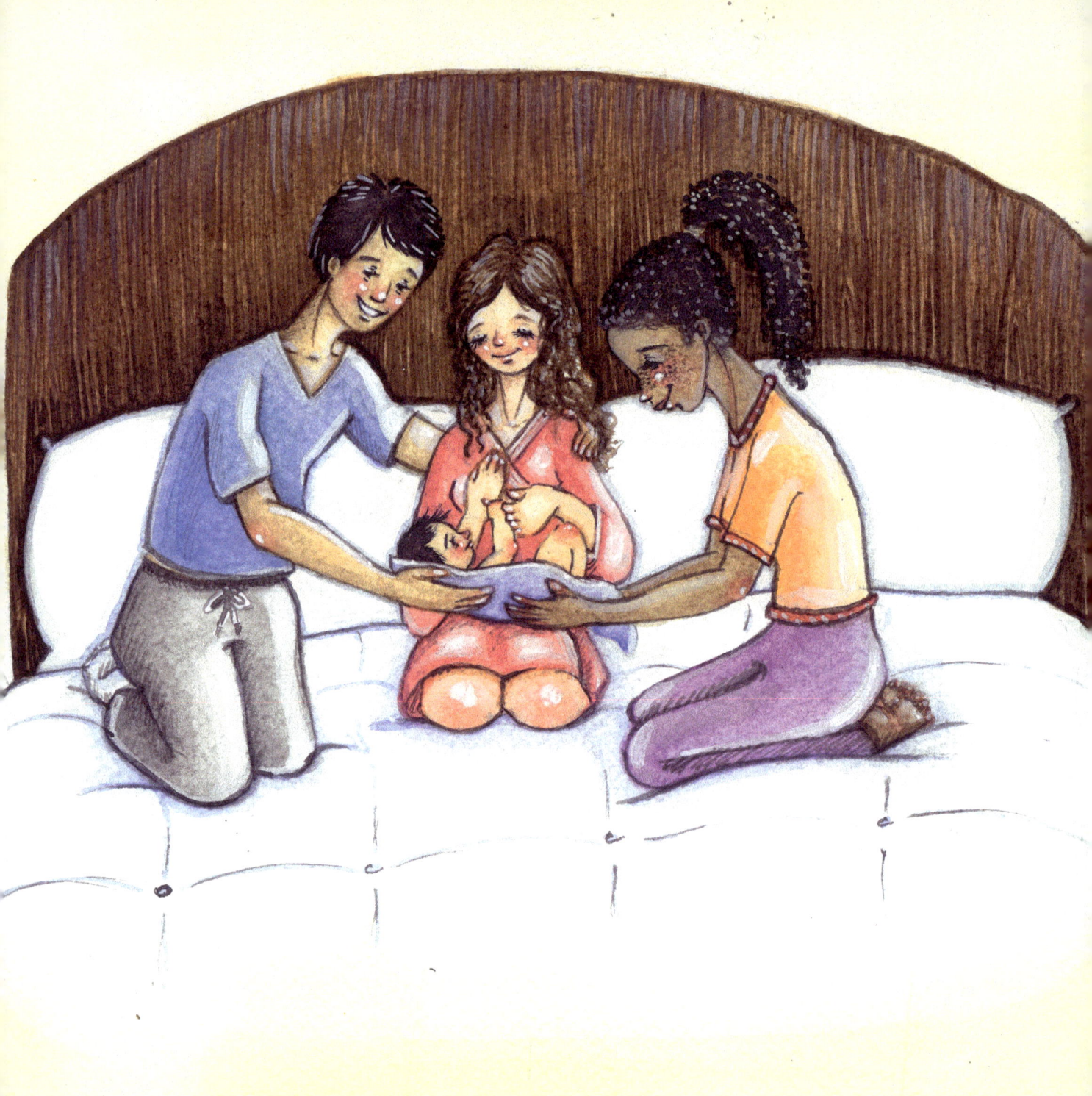

CHAPTER 11

Delivering Your Baby

This chapter covers perhaps one of the most important topics in this book: labor. I divided it into three parts. Part One covers Bella's birth, which was beautiful and far from ordinary. My hope is that you will be inspired to have a similar experience. Part Two helps you create your birth plan by taking you through five important questions and presenting your alternatives. Part Three offers comparison tables to complement your decision-making process.

Part One: Labor

The day before the marathon—signs that the baby is coming! I was a day short of 40 weeks on the day before Bella was born. It was an atypical day, and in retrospect, I should have seen her birth coming. I felt so tired and sleepy that I took two naps that day. I never felt that tired, but my body was asking me for rest that day because it was storing up energy for labor.

I began doing my routine workout video that evening and realized that I was modifying almost every move. I had been working out throughout my entire pregnancy in preparation for giving birth, but something *felt different*, and I didn't want to force myself that night. So, I turned off the TV and went to visit my grandmother, Andrea, with my oldest kids Abi and John. It was a wonderful day.

It was late by the time we got home. I realized it was past midnight when I took a shower and was getting ready for bed. That meant I was officially 40 weeks pregnant. So, I took a pregnancy pic before going to bed. Only five percent of babies born naturally are born on their due date. Most are born either a week before or after their due date. So, I was not expecting for my water to break just three hours later.

Most marathoners will tell you they rest the day before a big race. The same is true in preparation for labor. Bella may have been born earlier, before her time, if I would have pushed myself that day. Maybe her birth wouldn't have been so natural then.

It is important to help our body by listening to its cues and acting accordingly. This is particularly true and impactful during pregnancy and in leading up to labor. All of the organs, systems, and tissues are connected—your body knows what to do. This is why I think it is unhealthy to force your body into labor under normal circumstances. We go against our body's natural ways when we push ourselves into labor before our body's natural time. Your baby will come when he or she is ready.

When your water breaks. I woke up because of a strong contraction at 4:05 AM. I reached for my cell phone and tracked it on an app called Full Term—Contraction Timer. The contraction lasted ten minutes and was not going away, so I told JC and walked over to the bathroom to see if using the bathroom would make me feel better. I felt water running down my right leg on my way there. I checked to make sure it was amniotic fluid and it was! That meant that the amniotic sac where the baby was in had ruptured, and I would soon be in labor.

The water doesn't always break. As a matter of fact, most times it doesn't break until right before the baby is born. Sometimes your water breaks and contractions start coming right away. Other times your water breaks and contractions don't start coming until several hours later. Sheila, my midwife, showed us to use the acronym T.A.C.O. and advised us to call her with the following information if the water did break. (See **Table 11.1**).

JC called Sheila to let her know my water broke. We went over T.A.C.O. and everything was okay.

TABLE 11.1 EVALUATING AMNIOTIC FLUID

T	Time it broke.
A	Amount that came out—a gush versus a trickle.
C	Color—anything other than clear could indicate that your baby has passed meconium (bowel contents) while still in utero, which could increase baby's risk of infection.
O	Amniotic fluid should be odorless. An odor could indicate infection.

I drank coconut water because of its many electrolytes, but water is good too. Drinking plenty of fluids will keep your body energized and will replenish the amniotic fluid, which is particularly important if your water breaks. Urinating frequently will relax your muscles and help with labor.

Laboring. Both of my childbirths were beautiful, but each was different. Every labor is unique. Labors don't start the same, go the same, or end the same. None is just like the other. Don't feel like you need to labor like anyone else or like you did previously. Each birth is the beginning of a new story. So, be creative!

Don't be afraid to take the lead. You can follow the midwife's advice, but nobody knows about your needs better than you. Midwives are used to letting the body do its thing. The woman is in the lead, and the midwife is there to ensure safety. Feel free to be in your tub or the bed or even walking around.

I tried to go to sleep when my water broke with Bella. It is just like the beginning of a race when you make sure to pace yourself. The idea is to save your energy in the beginning of the race, despite the excitement, so that you don't burn out later on. The adrenaline and endorphins may drive you to go faster than your body can handle and that may result in an injury and stop you from being able to finish the race. Consider resting in the very beginning when you go into labor. Sometimes sleep is what your body needs to continue with the birthing process. This is especially helpful when labor isn't progressing.

Thankfully, I rested the day before, because I was so excited from my water breaking that I was only able to rest for about an hour between contractions. I let JC know when a contraction started and ended, and he tracked them for me. This is how we could tell if I was in active labor, or 5-1-1, which meant contractions were coming no more than five minutes apart, lasting at least one minute each, for over one hour. After one hour, we saw I was indeed in active labor, so we called Sheila again to let her know that she could come over.

I took a shower and got ready for an awesome day. I occasionally peeked out of the shower and told JC how happy I was. I even put on a little bit of make up in between contractions because I wanted to look nice in the pictures.

Natural birthing brings strong sensations you may have never felt before. You will appreciate how the contractions begin softly and increase in intensity as your baby approaches because you get to feel them from beginning to end. You can identify that you are in labor by monitoring your contractions if your labor begins without your water breaking. You may notice they are consistent in length and regularity during labor. As labor progresses, they can range from a menstrual cramping sensation, to stronger fiery cramps with back-pressure, to significantly more intense ones that may be difficult to describe. Some contractions are focused in the low abdominal area, others are in the back, and others are all over. Keeping your eyes closed and focusing on breathing deeply during contractions may help you during labor.[1]

JC saw the contractions were intensifying, and he called Dr. Lisa, my chiropractor, so she could come and help me as my doula.[2] We also planned on having our moms present during the birth, so I asked him to give them a heads up.

Dr. Lisa arrived very quickly. She offered to do a technique to ease the contractions and asked me to go on my bed on my elbows and knees. She performed a technique to relax my abdominal muscles, and it seemed to make the contractions better.

Sheila arrived shortly after. I was so excited that I gave her a tour of the house, forgetting I had already done so two weeks earlier during her home visit. I offered them coconut water and something to eat. I just went off to the side whenever a contraction hit and supported my body on a chair until the contraction went away. Sheila saw me in such good spirits that she was sure I wasn't going to be pushing anytime soon. She came with her assistant, but her assistant decided to leave when they saw my stamina.

Transitioning. It was 10:00 AM and I was hanging out in my kitchen with my family, Sheila, and Dr. Lisa. All of them were part of my birthing team and I felt very supported around them. I wasn't hungry, but Sheila told me I should have some carbs so that I had energy to push later on—so I had a banana and some toast. A first-time mom may labor for 10-20 hours, so light eating is a good practice to ensure she is energized throughout the labor. I paused whenever a contraction hit, let the contraction pass, and then resumed my conversation with them.

Contractions were coming regularly ever since my water broke six hours earlier. They were manageable and felt like strong menstrual cramps. It was not like what movies or TV shows typically portray. It was a very calm and happy environment.

As the contractions continued increasing in intensity, I found myself separating from my team and focusing on breathing through the contractions on my own. But JC was by my side all along. He was perfect. He did not say anything, but I knew I had his support and that he was right there for me if I needed anything.

I was using the bathroom when I suddenly threw up much of the coconut water and the breakfast that I had enjoyed earlier. I hadn't thrown up in years before that day, so it was very strange to me. JC let Sheila know what had happened,

and she said it was normal and that it was a sign that labor was progressing.[3]

JC was very nice and told me not to worry about it. He cleaned it and helped me get to the shower so that I could clean up. I felt very in tune with my body. A strong contraction hit while I was in the shower so I had to kneel on the shower floor to endure it and that position made it manageable.

When JC saw me on the floor, he asked me if I wanted to get in the bathtub. I didn't want to, so I told him I was okay and that the water in the tub from earlier was old and cold. It was hard for him to see me on the floor like that, so he insisted. I figured it was better than the floor, so I agreed and he quickly refilled it with hot water until the temperature was perfect. I am so glad he insisted because getting in the tub was very soothing. The water relaxed me and it was easier to endure the contractions even though they were stronger, longer, and the breaks in between them were shorter.

I switched positions until I found the one that made me feel better, which was on my hands and knees, swaying my hips side to side. Then,

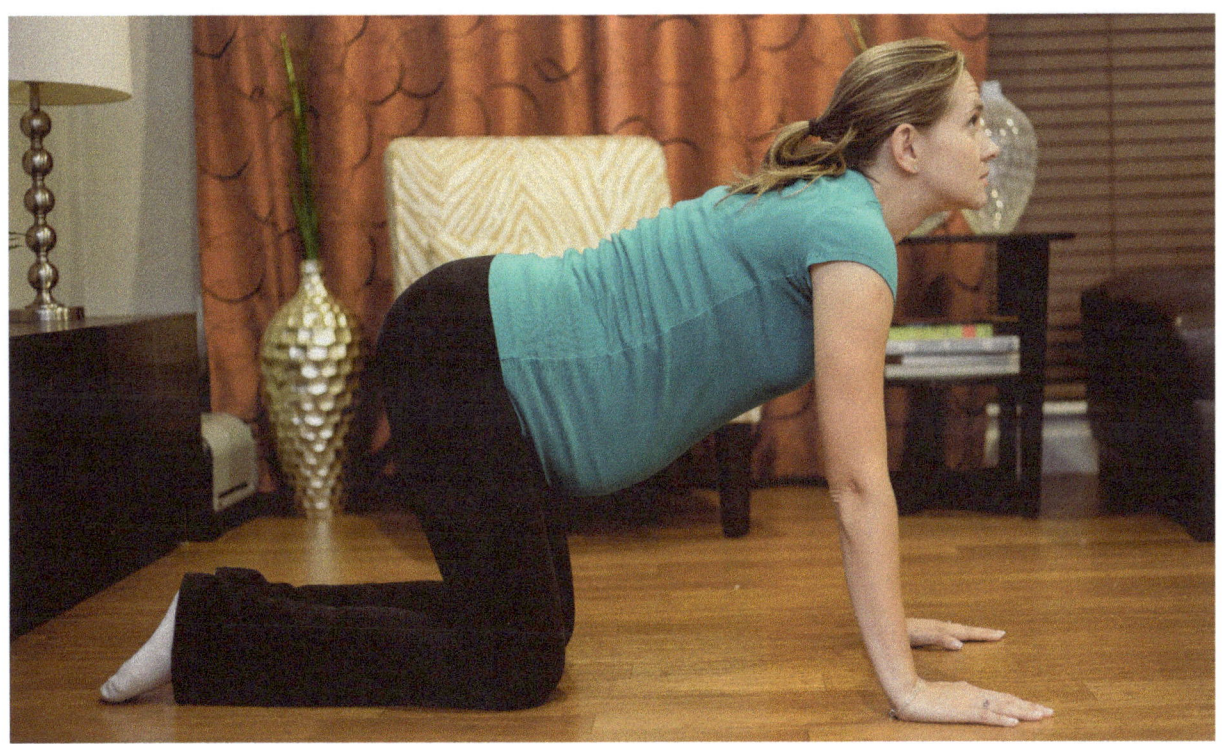

the contractions began feeling like heat surges that would come and go like waves crashing into the shoreline. I made sure to keep my cool in the midst of it all, breathing deeply and slowly with my eyes closed, just like Sharain, my birth instructor, taught me. I knew screaming or being loud wouldn't help Bella or myself. Instead, I saved my energy for the moment I had to push.

I wondered how much longer I was going to feel this way. I asked JC to get Sheila during a break from a contraction and asked her if she could check how dilated I was. Sheila didn't like to check dilation after the water broke to prevent infections and having the mom stressing about a number, but I really wanted her to check mine. I wanted to know how much longer this was going to last.

I noticed that Sheila made an effort to keep her composure when she checked me. And I thought that I might not be dilated enough when I saw her hesitate. *Maybe she doesn't want to disappoint me*, I thought. Birth is about endurance. I knew it wasn't a sprint, and I wasn't expecting it to be fast or easy. Then Sheila said, "Maria, give me your hand," in her usual gentle tone. My heart raced at the sound of her voice, and I was filled with excitement. She held my hand and gently stretched it out. I reached down and felt Bella's head. My baby was right there! And this marathon that we rightly so call *labor* was almost over!

Pushing. It is time to push. You can feel it all and there is no turning back. It feels like a huge amount of pressure in your anus. Almost like you are constipated and have to poop a big one. This is your baby, and that urge is your body telling you it's time to push. You are likely to be having a contraction at this time. Use that contraction to help you push. If you don't have a contraction, you can wait until you begin having one to push. The contractions are your helpers. Don't try to ignore them. Instead, accept the sensations that come with them. Embrace them. They are helping your baby come out. You will see that when you do, things will begin moving more easily and rapidly.

This is the most intense part of labor, but it also feels very relieving once it's over. Relaxing as much as you can when you are pushing and following your instincts to know how much and when to push will make a difference. You may feel the baby's head in the front of your vaginal opening and toward your anus as he or she approaches. Then, you may feel a burning sensation when the baby's head is coming out. Some call it "*the ring of fire.*" This is caused by your skin stretching to fit the baby's head. The stinging may mean that your skin is splitting. Control the way you push in order to sub-

side the sting and prevent tearing and possibly stitches. Unlike blowing a balloon too fast and popping it, imagine blowing it slowly and steadily. You can take a break when you feel the sting and pause until another contraction comes or you feel that you can push again. One of the many benefits of birthing in water is that it significantly reduces the risk of tearing. (See Chapter 8 for tips on how to prevent tearing).

The Birth. I asked JC to get the kids and our moms when I realized that Bella was right there so they could all see her birth. Dr. Lisa came right away and helped put cold compresses on my forehead to refresh me and prepare me for pushing. I asked JC to put worship music in the background. I hadn't planned on doing that, but I felt like I needed to. I was so happy and grateful that God was allowing me to experience my much-desired natural birth. I couldn't believe it was actually going to happen!

I told Sheila, "I want to push," as Hillsong music played in the background and I felt refreshed and energized. Sheila responded slowly, in her supportive tone, "Then, push." And just like that, I pushed. No one told me when to start or how long to push for. They didn't need to. I just had to tune into my body and follow its lead. It was very calm and peaceful. No chaos. Just beauty.

I could hear JC, my mom, and mother in law saying that I could do it and they could see Bella. Even my son John, who was seventeen at the time, said softly, "You can do it, mom." My aunt Gladys, who flew from Puerto Rico, was with us too. Having them with me was so encouraging. I pushed a second time and Bella's head came out. I couldn't see it, but I felt it.

Sheila checked to make sure that Bella's neck didn't have the umbilical cord around it and said, "The next push the baby is out." So, I gave one last push, and she asked JC if he wanted to "catch our baby" as Bella's body started coming out. This was exactly what we wanted. Bella's body came out completely and he received her and put her on my chest. They weren't kidding about those happy hormones that you feel when birthing naturally. I was ecstatic. It was the birth of my dreams!

In retrospect, my labor with Bella was so much more than the accomplishment of my much-desired natural birth. It was an empowering and life-changing experience. Birth stories like ours aren't very common, but they can be. I'm used to hearing comments like, "You were just made to give birth." But I truly believe that it has little to do with genetics and a lot more to do with a few decisions JC and I made in preparation for our daughter's birth. It all begins with a healthy pregnancy, but making sure you have the right birth plan is just as important.

Part Two: Creating the Right Birth Plan

Sheila, my midwife, gave me the best advice I can give you for determining your birth plan, "Follow your instincts. If you do, you won't have regrets." You can apply this advice to anything in your life, but especially when it comes to caring for your baby.

I gave my birth plan a lot of thought because it was important to me that Bella and I had the best environment for a natural birth and her first day of life. It is so important to think about what you want that day to be like. I like how Dr. Hernandez explains it, "As parents, we meticulously research the best day care, school, and baby sitter for our kids, but what about their first day in this world?" I'll add to that and say that during our pregnancies, we give so much thought to our baby's name, we research the best car seat, stroller, crib, and so many other things, but we settle for the status quo when it comes to the baby's birth. I encourage you to think about what you want your baby's birth to be like. Whatever decision you make, let it be a well thought out decision. Your baby's birth deserves more of your time than all the aforementioned things combined! So, let's create a plan to make that possible.

Create your birth plan by considering the following questions:

» Who will deliver your baby?
» Where will you deliver your baby?
» Who is on your birthing team?
» What interventions are you comfortable with?
» What protocol is important to you?

Who Will Deliver Your Baby?

One of the most important things to consider when creating your birth plan is who will be the right practitioner for your baby's birth. If you are passionate about experiencing a quick, drug-free, and natural birth, please know that your OB/GYN is not your only choice or your best option.

OB/GYNs are a good choice for high-risk births or women who want to have a C-section or have an epidural. An OB/GYN is the best choice for pregnant women with pre-existing health conditions or a problem with the baby's health. However, if you are in a low-risk and healthy pregnancy and want to have a natural birth, you will benefit from prenatal care and labor with a midwife.

Midwives are natural birth experts. Unlike many doctors who may perform more C-sections than vaginal births, midwives help women birth naturally every day. This is their daily bread. This is what they do. A midwife is trained to do everything an OB/GYN is trained to do with the exception of surgery.

Dr. Jeffrey Ecker is a professor of obstetrics, gynecology, and reproductive biology, a high-risk Obstetrician at Massachusetts General Hospital, and the Director of his department's quality and safety program. He says that if you have a low-risk population of pregnant women, a "great model" might be "to have midwives providing uncomplicated prenatal care and doing all the uncomplicated deliveries," while a few doctors focus on problem cases and perform C-sections.[4]

Prenatal care with a midwife tends to be more personal and the treatment options are more natural. This was important to me based on my recommendations in Chapter 8. When I found out I was pregnant with Bella, I first went to my OB/GYN. At that time, I didn't know I had other options. It wasn't until later, after Dr. Lisa interviewed Sheila, that I transferred my care to a midwife. A glucose test with a midwife consisted of eating a particular heavy meal, but my OB/GYN didn't give that option and I ended up drinking a sugary juice that gave me the jitters.

When I found out I was pregnant with Mila, I also first went to my OB/GYN, since she was closer to home. I thought I could manage the typical interventions until I was further in my pregnancy. Although I was able to get away from the use of ultrasounds, my OB/GYN was very persuasive in using the doppler. Once I transferred to Sheila we used a fetoscope, which does not use sound waves and its safety is indisputable.

Today, professional midwives are responsible for attending women during labor and childbirth in much of the world. In fact, midwives are the primary care providers to pregnant women in the countries with the best pregnancy outcomes. Popular pregnancy books state that the hospital is the safest place for delivering your baby. I disagree, and the statistics support my opinion. World Health Organization statistics show that births attended by midwives have lower infection rates, lower C-section rates, fewer complications, and healthier outcomes—thus, lower overall medical costs—than physician-attended hospital births.[5] In addition, there is no difference in infant mortality rates between midwife-attended and physician-attended births for low-risk women. Countries such as the Netherlands, Sweden, and New Zealand, which have the best birth outcome statistics in the world, use midwives as their main maternity care providers.[6]

Bringing it back to our roots. Midwives have been delivering babies for ages, even before recorded history. The earliest references to midwives appear on Egyptian scrolls dating back to 1500–1900 B.C. The midwife is even mentioned in the *Bible* in Genesis 35:17 and in Exodus 1:20. In 1900, midwives attended half of the births in the U.S., and only about five percent of births happened in hospitals.

Even though midwifery may seem distant to some, women shifted from midwives and home births to doctors and hospitals only a few decades ago. Perhaps this is why one-third of American babies are born by C-section. Most U.S. experts—whether high-risk obstetricians or home-birth midwives—agree that the U.S. rate is higher than medically necessary and acknowledge that many women are undergoing major surgery for avoidable reasons.

According to the U.S. Department of Health and Human Services, 85% of American pregnancies achieve full term without complications. That's a figure that many midwives believe Americans often lose sight of. They say that simply seeing pregnancy and birth as normal, rather than as a medical problem, would help lower the C-section rate. Dr. Ecker says that his patients, too, are influenced by tales, including the tragedies on television, the co-worker's near miss, and/or the warnings online. According to Dr. Ecker, patients often focus on the numerator (the very rare cases) rather than on the denominator (the great majority for whom everything goes well).[7]

An easy way to prevent a C-section. Janet Singer, a midwife who teaches medical students and residents at Women & Infants Hospital of Rhode Island in Providence, explains that "failure to progress" is perhaps the most-preventable reason for cesareans. "Failure to progress" is when a provider decides that labor is proceeding too slowly to be safe. According to a year 2000 study in *Obstetrics and Gynecology*, diagnoses of failure to progress rose along with the C-section rate in the twentieth century from 3.8% in 1970, to 11.6% in 1989, and to 16.1% by 1995.[8] Unlike an OB/GYN, who has the C-section option readily available, a midwife will try everything in her scope to help you birth naturally. Midwives are also far more tolerant of slow labors and are therefore less likely to diagnose the need for a C-section under these circumstances.

VBACs. Midwives can also perform a VBAC (vaginal birth after caesarean or "trial of labor") so you can have a natural birth even after a previous C-section. VBACs are very common all around the world. With a success rate of 99.5%, this means that only .5% of uteruses will rupture. Out of that .5%, the most common is the asymptomatic rupture, which the baby can survive.

Unfortunately, attempting VBACs in a hospital setting has become rare, with successful ones even rarer. "We know from studies that what increases your chances of having a VBAC are things like not having epidural anesthesia and being up and moving about and having continuous labor support," says Dr. Cara Osborne.[9] "But because, in many practitioners' minds, the trial of labor is unlikely to work, they're setting up for a surgical scenario." Hospitals may encourage or even require a woman to use epidural anesthesia during labor, she explains, "because they want to have it on board if she has a C-section." In addition, hospitals usually require continuous fetal monitoring in the form of wires attached to the laboring woman's abdomen, which restricts mobility. As Dr. Osborne points out, "The things that would help someone have a successful VBAC are often things that are not offered to her because the assumption is that this is likely to end in another C-section."[10]

Breech deliveries. In 2006, the American Congress of Obstetricians and Gynecologists (ACOG) changed its position on the need for a caesarean in the case of a breech, stating that a clinician with sufficient experience and support might appropriately assist in vaginal breech deliveries. Midwives will deliver a breech baby, yet obstetricians prefer to perform a C-section. "Doctors perform cesareans, in part, because they aren't trained to favor or perform less-invasive techniques. With inadequate training and experience, liability and patient risk increases. Thus, few hospitals even offer the option of vaginal breech delivery."[11]

What to look for in a midwife. It is very important to find a midwife that is right for you. When Dr. Lisa, my chiropractor and doula, heard that I wanted a natural birth she said she would interview a few midwives and let me know which ones she liked. I trusted Dr. Lisa and knew she would only recommend the one that met her highest standards. This is how I got to my midwife, Sheila Simms Watson. When I first called her, she told me she was booked and that I may prefer a midwife closer to home because she was about 30 minutes away, but I told her I wanted to meet with her because she was highly recommended. Dr. Lisa also gave me the contact to another midwife, but I didn't feel the connection I felt with Sheila when we spoke on the phone. The feeling you get with your midwife is very important.

I felt an immediate connection with Sheila. Several days later, she called me to tell me that she had a spot for me because a woman changed her mind about birthing in Florida. I was so happy. JC and I immediately made an appointment to meet her. I was further motivated and empowered when I met her in person. We chose Sheila for a few reasons, but primari-

ly because of her natural and holistic approach. Sheila had 20 years of experience under her belt, no casualties and only two postpartum hospital transfers, and she had even delivered breech babies.

When JC and I interviewed her, she made us feel comfortable. She answered all of our questions and put our doubts to ease. We both liked her personality very much. She was evidently very knowledgeable.

Table 11.2 includes the questionnaire Dr. Lisa used to interview the midwives. I hope this helps you find the perfect midwife (or practitioner) for you.

Here are additional considerations:

- Years of experience—evaluate if it is a number that you are comfortable with.
- How long can a woman be in labor for? A woman can labor for days. Look for signs that she evaluates the baby's and

TABLE 11.2: MIDWIFE INTERVIEW QUESTIONS

Category	Question	Considerations
Birth Overview	Tell me about a typical birth.	Is this the kind of birth you want to have?
Hospital Transfer	When do you think a transport is necessary and how often does it happen?	If the midwife delivers at home, this means what percentage of her deliveries end up at the hospital. The number should be closer to 5% and in no case more than 50%. Just like you would ask your doctor for his/her C-section rate, ask your midwife for her stats on hospital transfers. My midwife has only transferred twice in 23 years of experience. Both times were after the baby was born because the placenta wouldn't deliver.
Time to Birth	How long do you allow a mother to labor at home after the water breaks? How long are you comfortable with?	Look for discernment and leeway.
Interventions	Do you use a doppler or a stethoscope?	The effects of dopplers on your baby are not all known. A stethoscope or fetoscope is a more natural method. More information on the safety of Dopplers and ultrasounds is found in Chapter 8.
Delivering Your Baby	How much do you assist in bringing the baby out?	They check that the baby's neck is free from the umbilical cord. She should avoid pulling the neck and allow the baby to come out on his or her own.
Umbilical Cord	How long do you wait before cutting the umbilical cord?	You should let the cord finish pulsating before cutting it or wait until the placenta is delivered.

mom's well being and that she promotes nourishment and resting in intervals to keep mom steady and healthy.

- Does she have a page with reviews or videos?
- How does she evaluate labor as far as progression? She observes the frequency and intensity of contractions. She lets the mom labor without the pressure of dilation and a ticking clock. She considers if the membranes ruptured and any symptoms such as nausea or diarrhea, which are common during Transition.
- How does she help labor progress? Look for specific methods, such as nipple stimulation.
- Ask about any casualties. Sheila had never had a casualty. This was important to me.
- Discuss protocol—look for mom-led and freedom to let breastfeeding occur within the first hour.
- Could she be your friend? How does she make you feel? When you birth at home, your midwives are there to support you throughout your labor and baby's birth—not just for a few minutes at a time every few hours, as in a hospital setting. Evaluate your compatibility. The better your relationship with your midwife, the easier it will be to work together through your pregnancy and labor. Communicate any concerns you have throughout your prenatal care so that there is transparency between you two. Trust is very important in this relationship.

Back-Up Plan. I planned for my OB/GYN, Dr. Monica Daniel, to be my back-up doctor in case labor did not progress at home. Dr. Daniel had been my OB/GYN for many years. She was supportive of my desire to birth at home. When I asked her to be my back up doctor, she agreed. Our plan was for her to deliver my baby if she was on call and for another OB/GYN from her practice to do it if she was unavailable. This way I wouldn't end up with just any doctor. You should interview your backup doctor just like you interview your midwife. Find out his or her statistics on C-sections.

Where Will You Deliver Your Baby?

If you deliver with an OB/GYN, your choice will most likely be limited to the hospital that your doctor delivers in. I know there are doctors who deliver at home in places like Costa Rica or Puerto Rico. But it is most common to deliver in a hospital if you are under the care of an OB/GYN. If you are using a midwife, you have the choice of delivering in a hospital, a birthing center, or at home.

Throughout my pregnancy with Bella, I watched different reality shows on childbirth and was disturbed that most of them ended up in C-sections. It all made sense when I watched the documentary *The Business of Being Born*.[12] I knew the hospital was not the place for me because I wanted a natural birth. I wanted to be as far away from all drugs as possible and I wanted to be on my turf. I felt a home birth would facilitate birthing naturally and a hospital environment would make that harder for me.

I didn't always plan on having a home birth. We initially wanted a natural birth at a hospital, but were disappointed when we went on a tour of the reputable and state-of-the-art hospital we were considering and saw that the "natural birth suite" didn't look very different from a normal room, with the exception of some minor décor. They told me that the nurses in those rooms were more pro-natural birth and supportive, but the cold room, bright lights, and funky smell of the hospital were enough to turn me off.

I then heard many stories of women who were trying to birth naturally in natural suites at the hospital and were offered an epidural multiple times. One of my friends told me, "It felt like every time I was having a tough contraction a nurse would come in and offer an epidural. The last thing they told me was that if I wanted one I would have to get it now because the anesthesiologist was leaving." I have heard this happen to other women too. They were told the anesthesiologist was leaving and were pressured into getting the epidural right away out of fear that it would not be available later.

I knew I didn't want to birth at a hospital. At a hospital, you are on their turf and they can really make you feel like it. I didn't want to be bossed around or rushed if I wasn't giving birth by a certain time. I didn't want my baby to be taken away from me after giving birth. I didn't want people making these decisions for me.

A natural birth is possible in a hospital setting as well, but know that you will be going against the flow. If you want to have a hospital birth, know that it won't necessarily be easy even if you are in a natural birthing room. An important tip is to be up front with your decisions. *Tell the doctor your plan* and make sure he or she writes it on your file. *Communicate your birth plan* to the hospital staff. They will offer you an epidural even though you are in a natural birthing room. *Designate a person you trust to look out for the fulfillment of your birth plan.* You will be busy breathing through your contractions, and someone else can make a decision that is not in accordance with your birth plan. This is not rare. The hospital staff may make decisions without consulting you, thinking it is for your well-being. Make sure this person is watching what the staff does in regards to your care and another person is looking out for the baby once he or she is born. Research your odds. Look at your doctor's stats. Look at your hospital's stats. If you want a natural birth and most of your doctor's births are C-sections, then consider switching to a doctor that does mostly natural births. And don't just take their word for it—ask for a report.

Women who are high-risk or want to use pain management medication during labor are good candidates for a hospital birth. But the hospital is not your best environment if you *really* want a natural and drug free birth. When I first learned about home births from one of my best friends Samantha C., I thought it was a crazy idea. But after becoming pregnant with Bella and researching my options, I realized that birthing at home was safe and the best way to have a natural birth. I had no idea what contractions felt like. I only knew what others had told me about them and what I read in many birthing books. But no matter how "hard" or "painful" they may be, I was certain without any degree of doubt of one thing: I wanted to give birth *at home*.

There were two things in my birth plan that were most important to me: birthing naturally and having a safe environment for my baby on her first day of life. I wanted to experience giving birth in a calm and peaceful environment: able to breathe through my contractions without any distractions, walking around freely, eating if I was hungry and drinking if I was thirsty, giving birth to my daughter Bella in water surrounded by my family, and doing it all in the comfort of my home.

I love my home. I am comfortable in there. It is my turf. My bed is my favorite place in my home. Just imagining I would be in the most comfortable place for me during labor just made sense. I also wanted Bella's birth to be peaceful and beautiful, and my home was the perfect place to achieve that.

If you decide to birth at home, take advantage of your freedom. You are not allowed to eat or drink at the hospital. At home, you can. You can watch a movie on your favorite couch or go for a walk around your neighborhood. Standing up as much as possible during labor will speed up the process, so this important.

Nesting. You may have an urge to clean and organize your home in preparation of your baby's arrival. This desire is a normal part of pregnancy called "nesting." It may be more intense if you plan to birth at home and may increase as your due date approaches. Nesting may be a very healthy form of exercise. Prepare your home in advance to make sure you are comfortable the day of your baby's birth. I had three clear bins that contained all the birthing supplies and baby's needs for the first few days. I numbered the bins and had a list indicating what was inside each bin. This made it easy for my midwife and team to readily find whatever they needed. I also deep-cleaned my home, and even labeled my utensils drawer! I can laugh about it now.

A water birth. You can have a water birth at home, a birthing center, and some hospitals. Water births make contractions more manageable and reduce the risk of perineum tears.

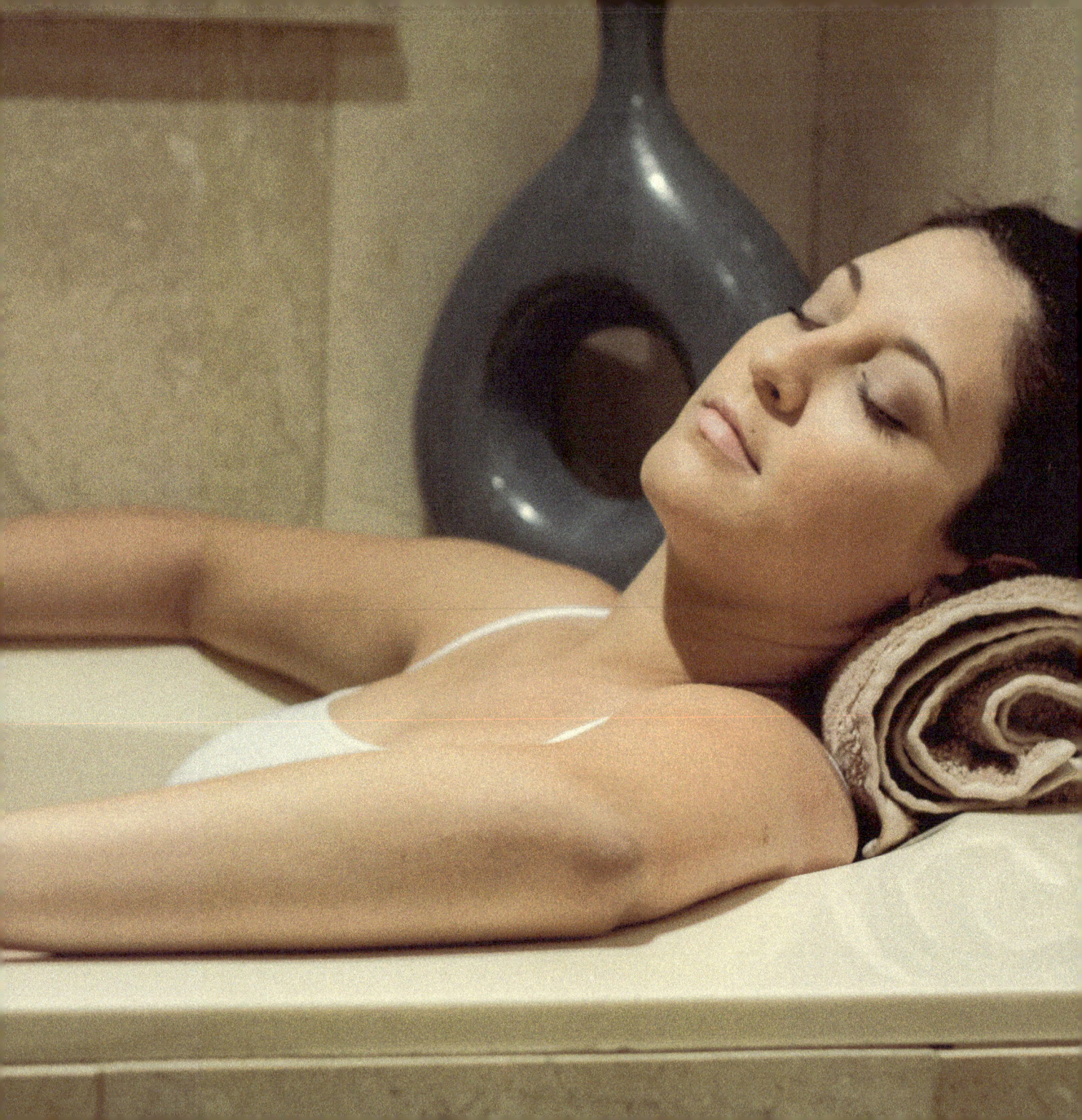

My midwife, Sheila, explains the benefits behind birthing in water.

"Water birth" is the use of a heated water bath or pool by a laboring woman during labor and birth. Most people are drawn to water. Few things feel better than a soak in the tub after a hard day's work. Water becomes even more desirable during pregnancy, labor, and birth. Perhaps this basic familiarity stays with us because we begin our lives in the womb surrounded by liquid.

Women have been using water to ease labor and facilitate birth for thousands of years. Many women report a sensation like an "energy surge" that moves through them as soon as they step into water. When a woman in labor relaxes in a warm tub, free from gravity's pull on her body, with sensory stimulation reduced, her body is less likely to secrete stress-related hormones. This allows her body to produce the pain inhibitors (endorphins) that complement labor.

Women achieve a level of comfort in water that, in turn, reduces their levels of fear and stress. Women's perception of pain is greatly influenced by their level of anxiety. When labor becomes physically easier, a woman's ability to concentrate calmly is improved and she is able to focus inward on the birth processes. Water helps some women reach a state of consciousness in which their fear and resistance are diminished or removed completely; their bodies then relax, and their babies are born in the easiest, most gentle way possible.

The ease of the mother who labors and gives birth in water becomes the ease of the child who is born in the water. The baby has been in amniotic water through pregnancy, and being born in water is a gentle transition from the womb to your loving arms. Water is familiar to the baby and helps him or her feel more secure. The baby emerges into the water and is "caught" either by the mother, father, or the birth attendant. In the water, the child has freedom of movement within familiar fluid surroundings. A baby's limbs can also unfold with greater ease during those first moments when leaving the mother's body and entering the water. The water offers a familiar comfort after the stress of birth, reassuring the child and allowing the bodily systems time to organize.

Being in water also helps to soften the perineum and makes it easier to be born without tearing or needing an episiotomy, and therefore, no stitches."

Birthing at home is safe. I noticed how Sheila and her assistant became very focused on Bella's well-being from the moment she was born. They were checking her and making sure she was okay. Your midwife is there to ensure your safety and the baby's safety when birthing at home. You can also transfer to the nearest hospital at any point if she deems it necessary.

I remember telling a friend about my plan to birth at home when I was pregnant with Bella, and he told me that I was throwing away hundreds of years of progress. Just like him, many people think that the shift from home births to hospital births was progress and resulted in better maternal and infant mortality rates. However, that is not the case. These rates did not improve after shifting the main location of birth to the hospital.

I also considered a birthing center at one point. A midwife-led birthing center is a hybrid between the hospital and a home birth. It is ideal for people who want to be close to a hospital, but in a home-like environment. I knew a home birth was right for me when I learned that a midwife delivering at home brings and uses the same equipment available at a birthing center. We had a hospital nearby in the event we needed intervention.

You can deliver naturally at the hospital. My friend Carolina was pregnant with her first-born, Charlotte. She was fascinated by Bella's birth story and wanted a similar experience. She wanted a natural birth, but she didn't want to birth at home. I asked her to share her successful birth story with you.

I was attending my yearly holiday luncheon that day. I remember being so tired that I even wondered how I was going to make it home. I laid on my bed and took a nap once I arrived home. My bladder felt full when I got up about an hour later, so I went to the bathroom. I went back to bed, but it felt full once again. I tried to get back to the bathroom, but I couldn't make it. I felt like I was peeing on myself, but it was not pee. My water had broken.

I called my husband, John, and told him the baby was coming. The contractions began shortly after. The baby was early by one month, so I had not packed yet. I started packing until John got home and we finished together. I stopped every four minutes for my contractions, which lasted about thirty seconds. The pain was not very strong. It was manageable.

THE SECRETS TO A HEALTHY PREGNANCY

We called my sister while on our way to the hospital so that she could be there for the birth. John thought it would be helpful to have someone else helping too. I checked in at triage and was already five centimeters dilated. The staff asked me if I wanted an epidural. I asked John if he believed that I could do it without medicine and he said yes. So I declined, knowing that my husband was supporting me. I was five centimeters dilated by 10:00 PM and reached eight centimeters by midnight. John timed my contractions and looked at the monitor to tell me when the next contraction was coming, peaking, and ending. This was very helpful to me in managing the contractions and the pain.

John and my sister put together a playlist of Christian worship music that I liked. This was also very helpful when I needed to focus on something other than the contractions. The nurses were very helpful in making me comfortable. A nurse counted softly in my ear once I began to push so that I could hold my push. John was on my other ear encouraging me. My sister was praying for me the entire time. I was singing and praying for the hospital, the staff, and the doctors the entire time.

I pushed for one hour and Charlotte was finally born at 2:30AM. My sister was with me while John was with the baby and they took turns. I liked that the baby and I were never left alone. I really needed the support while they were stitching me up because I had no pain medicine. Afterwards, they attached Charlotte to my breast and she latched on immediately.

Who is on Your Birthing Team?

For Bella's birth, we called our midwife, Sheila, to let her know when my water broke. I liked that I didn't have to endure a ride to the hospital with contractions. Sheila came to guide us through it all. She arrived with a birth attendant, who left while I was laboring, but came back after Bella was born. I also called my chiropractor, Dr. Lisa, who acted as my doula, as you already know. We texted our older kids, Abi and John, to let them know they didn't have to go to school because their little sister was surely going to be born today. Then, when we realized I was in active labor, we called my mom and mother in law and asked them to come over. JC was by my side at all times. This was my birthing team. Unlike in the hospital, where I would have been birthing with nurses that I just met, or the number of family members in my birthing room may have been restricted, I was birthing at home with the people I love. I felt like everyone involved in Bella's birth was on my side and supporting me with my desires to birth naturally.

Sheila says that, "Being surrounded by the people and environment a woman enjoys most in her life helps maintain a positive outcome and keeps anxiety and fears to a minimum." Think about who you want to be there during your birth. Don't leave it up to chance. You are at a very vulnerable stage when you are giving birth. Make sure you select people who will bring out the best in you. Don't be afraid to exclude people who may hinder your labor. You can explain that you want to have the best chance at a natural birth and having many people around may be a distraction. They love you, and they will understand.

What Interventions are You Comfortable With?

I was in Puerto Rico, and the news that I was writing a book about pregnancy was out. I visited Lourdes, my esthetician, and she told me her daughter just had a baby and she shared her birth story. Lourdes has three children and birthed all of them naturally—even her eleven pound one—because she wanted to *feel* the birth. She wanted to know what it was like to push her baby, and she did not want a C-section.

So, it is not surprising that Lourdes' daughter also wanted a natural birth. She was so determined that she signed a form with her OB/GYN indicating her plan to abstain from drugs during labor. She labored in the hospital, and they offered something for the pain. In that moment, in the midst of the contractions, she accepted—not knowing that her daughter was about to be born. Lourdes says that her daughter was so groggy from the meds that she wasn't able to fully enjoy and experience the moment of her daughter's birth.

One of the main reasons I wanted to birth naturally was because my mom had me naturally. When I asked my mom why she chose a natural birth she said that she wanted me to be free from drugs. That made sense considering that an epidural is a drug and that all drugs have side effects.[13] At this point I have seen hundreds of births and read about another hundred birth stories. I found the most beautiful ones to be those where the mom was free to walk around and help her baby descend, drinking water if she was thirsty, eating if she was hungry, and surrounded by her family in the comfort of her home. Research shows that babies born through natural childbirth are more alert and show more interest in breastfeeding once delivered. For me, it was also important to experience birthing with all of my senses. I wanted to be alert and active.

Birth is a natural and normal process. Women have been birthing naturally for ages, but the use of interventions became normal when women began birthing in hospitals in the early 1900s. Hospitals used the twilight sleep to deliver babies in the 1930s. It put women in a state of partial narcosis without total loss of consciousness. This method of childbirth completely removed a mother from the birth experience, prevented her from being an agent in her own care, and the necessary isolation prevented the woman's family from advocating for her while she labored. American medical doctors also began a campaign against midwifery in the press, the courts, and in Congress around that time.

Hospitals use epidurals and sedatives among other drugs to make labor easier. But in reality, we make it harder and longer. Labor is often shorter when birthing naturally. Pain medications, including epidurals, often interfere with the body's natural way of laboring and can slow down contractions. Your body will guide you through birth when you don't interfere with its natural way. It knows what to do, and it is producing hormones that will help you dilate and birth your baby safely.

Chapter 7 covered how a chiropractor can turn a breech baby naturally without forcing the baby externally. Exercises and homeopathy can help the baby get in position if a baby is still breech around 34 weeks. I took 200c of homeopathic Pulsatilla once a day and did breech tilts for 10 minutes twice a day until Sheila confirmed that Bella turned. A breech tilt involves raising your pelvis. You can do this by propping it with pillows or laying on the floor and putting your feet on your bed so that your pelvis is 9 to 12 inches above your head.

However, there is a tendency for a baby to become breech *at the hospital* if an epidural is used. "Professor of obstetrics, gynecology, and reproductive biology, Ellice Lieberman, led a crucial study in 2005 that showed that epidural use increased the likelihood of an abnormally positioned baby at the time of delivery. Doctors already knew that the anesthetic made fever in labor more likely and tended to prolong labors. Lieberman's study showed that 'it's not that women are coming in and getting epidurals because their baby's in an abnormal position,' she says. Rather, babies were in [breech] position, in some cases, because of the epidural. The study found the position four times as often in women who used epidurals as in those who didn't—but no significant difference in frequency of abnormal position before the women had chosen the anesthesia."[14]

Many women will tell you the epidural was the most painful part of giving birth—even the ones whose epidural didn't work and had to push anyways. A woman can no longer walk around to help her baby descend after she receives an epidural. Instead, she is confined to her bed. This makes it harder for the baby to be born. The doctor may choose to add Pitocin to stimulate the uterus because labor may slow down after an epidural. Pitocin contractions are stronger and faster than natural contractions. There is very little recovery time between Pitocin contractions, leaving less oxygen to reach the baby.[15] The baby then to goes into distress, heartbeats decrease, and the doctor does an emergency C-section or a painful episiotomy. People think that the doctor saved the day, but in reality it could have all been avoided without any interventions in the first place.[16]

I've spoken to hundreds of women over the last three years who have shared with me about their pregnancies and births. I know many women who want to experience birthing naturally—not because they like pain, but because of they understand that interventions and medications don't come without a price. Many times, unfortunately, the price is not being able to experience a pleasant and memorable birth.

In a Harvard article on the rising rate of C-sections in the United States, Dr. Ecker says that whenever appropriate, physicians and patients should avoid interventions and prevent that "cascade" or snowball effect that that leads to a C-section.[17] He also asserts his respect for midwifery and includes that "our current legal environment reinforces this dynamic of cascading interventions since 'No one gets sued for doing a C-section,' obstetricians famously say. They do get sued for not intervening."

The Harvard article describes how the medical profession has increasingly sought to standardize care. Hospitals have come to require procedures that minimize the worst outcomes and can be easily regulated. Certain procedures, such as forceps deliveries, have waned because they are difficult to teach and perform. Fetal monitoring, which increases cesarean rates, has become established for overseeing and regulating care. And cesareans have increased because they are essential for preventing the worst outcomes and because they followed other interventions in some cases, they are relatively easy to teach and perform, and they are unlikely to provoke lawsuits.

I've heard from so many women who feel they got cheated out of their natural birth at the hospital because they were given Pitocin or an epidural, and that came with many consequences, most of them ending in a C-section. My fear of the drugs and ultimately a C-section was greater than my fear of contractions and pain.

You will experience different sensations during a contraction. They can range from a menstrual cramp sensation to very strong menstrual cramps accompanied by heat surges and back discomfort. When it gets stronger and you think you can't handle it, it means you are almost through with it. Remind yourself you can do it and that it is worth it. Every contraction brings you closer to holding your baby in your arms. This is what Ricki Lake calls "pain with purpose" in The Business of Being Born.[18]

Four of the major hormonal systems are active during labor and birth. These involve oxytocin, the hormone of love; endorphins, hormones of pleasure and transcendence; adrenaline and noradrenaline (epinephrine and norepinephrine), hormones of excitement; and prolactin, the mothering hormone.[19] Fluids administered directly into the bloodstream via an IV will dilute the body's natural chemistry. In addition, you cannot feel contractions and pushing instinctively becomes a lot harder when an epidural is administered. During Mila's quick birth, I found that pushing through a contraction made her descend faster. This would be difficult to do after an epidural.

Your body continues releasing endorphins after labor. This is your body's natural way of dealing with pain. Endorphins are the most natural form of pain-relief. They calm you and make you feel very good. Studies show endorphin levels are reduced when an epidural is used for pain relief.[20]

Make sure to take a natural birthing course if you choose to avoid interventions. I took the Birthing From Within course and I found it very helpful during labor. The most impacting thing that I learned was how to breathe through my contractions—always with my eyes closed and taking deep breaths. Also check Ina May's Guide to Childbirth book for inspiration. The first part of the book is filled with amazing natural birth stories. One of my favorite lessons learned from her book was that an open mouth and a relaxed jaw during labor translates into a more elastic cervix, vagina, and anus that can open to full capacity. She shares that women who are able to do this rarely need stitches after childbirth.[21]

What Protocol is Important to You?

There were a few things I wanted to make sure happened during and after the births of my daughters. First, I wanted for JC to "catch" or receive the baby right after she exited the birth canal while she was still in water. I felt this was something very special that both of them would treasure. Our midwife asked JC if he wanted to receive Bella when she was born—just like we planned. Thankfully, that was a good lesson because little did we know that he would single-handedly deliver Mila a couple of years later. JC was the first person to hold our daughters for

the very first time during both of our births. His hands were the first hands they felt when they entered this world. That was so special for him and for both of my daughters.

Another thing that was important to me was to get my baby right after birth and place her on my chest, skin to skin. Birth is a pretty tough experience for babies, and they get tired form it. He or she has gone through a lot and is now in this whole new world. Thankfully, the baby has you. You are your baby's comfort zone. He or she knows you, your voice, and your heartbeat more than anything else in this world. Placing your baby on your chest soothes and comforts the baby. It will calm the breathing and even help regulate it through his or her connection with yours as your chest comes up and down. Skin to skin immediately after birth also stabilizes and normalizes the baby's temperature, heart rate, and blood sugar.[22]

An article published by PubMed.gov studying the effects of skin to skin a year after birth supports the practice of skin to skin contact, early breastfeeding, or both during the first two hours after birth.[23] When compared with separation between the mothers and their infants, skin-to-skin positively affected the variables of a Parent-Child Early Relational Assessment, which tests maternal sensitivity, an infant's self-regulation, and dyadic mutuality and reciprocity at one year after birth. The negative effect of a two-hour separation after birth was not compensated for by the practice of rooming-in. These findings support the presence of a period after birth, the early "sensitive period," during which close contact between mother and infant may induce a long-term positive effect on mother-infant interaction. In addition, swaddling of the infant was found to decrease the mother's responsiveness to the infant, her ability for positive affective involvement with the infant, and the mutuality and reciprocity in the dyad.[24]

My midwife Sheila puts it this way: "The first kind of abuse that can be done unto a child is separating him or her from her mother right after birth." I wanted my baby to be given to me after birth, and I didn't want to have to fight with nurses and hospital staff for this. I understand hospitals have staff limitations and protocols to protect them from lawsuits. This is something you don't have to worry about at home.

The best time to establish breastfeeding is right after delivering your baby. Babies who are kept skin to skin with the mother immediately after birth for at least an hour are more likely to latch on without any help and they are more likely to latch on well, especially if the mother did not receive medication during the labor or birth.[25] We did the breast crawl once my babies were calm and stable. It involves putting the baby on the middle of your chest and letting him or her find the breast and begin nursing independently when he or she is ready. This is a natural way to establish breastfeeding, and doing it shortly after birth also maximizes your chances of successfully breastfeeding right away. It is a beautiful thing to see your newborn baby slowly move his or her head, evidently knowing exactly where the milk is, and latch on enthusiastically when arriving at your breast.

Breastfeeding before the placenta is out naturally facilitates its delivery. This is called the third stage of labor. Your body is creating oxytocin while you are breastfeeding and that helps your uterus contract. These contractions will facilitate the delivery of your placenta. Your body is also pulsating blood into your baby through the umbilical cord during this time. Cutting the cord prematurely would only rob your baby of valuable and empowering cord blood cells that will surely make him or her a healthier adult.

The cord can be cut once the placenta is delivered. I wanted JC to do the honors. Cutting the umbilical cord is a special moment. The umbilical cord is what has been nourishing your baby for 40 weeks—his or her entire life so far. The placenta and the cord have been your baby's support for oxygen and for food. Cutting the cord is symbolic for the baby no longer being dependent on the placenta because he or she has you. Letting the father cut the cord makes him a part of that. Birth is very mom-centric, and including dad in these special moments will make it very memorable for both of you. Also note that your loved one can request to cut the umbilical cord at most hospitals and can even wait until the umbilical cord stops pulsating to do so.

I also wanted to do cord blood banking with both Bella and Mila, so the birth attendant collected the remaining cord blood cells and tissue after I delivered the placenta. We didn't have enough cell count in either to guarantee that it would be enough in the unlikely and undesired event that we would need it in the future because we let the blood pulsate during both births. I was okay with that because that meant both of my babies received the cord blood right after birth. Thus, they will be stronger throughout their whole life. We decided to donate the cells and keep the cord blood tissue for Mila's birth. You can go to *www.viacord.com* for more information on cord and tissue banking. After doing much research, I found them to be the best company for this service.

After Bella's birth, I came out of the water after delivering the placenta and my team helped me get to my bed where fresh new sheets awaited me. I felt euphoric. It was a feeling of extreme happiness. I lay down and saw how they checked and weighed my baby. Contractions continued coming irregularly after delivery and, for a couple of days, decreased in intensity, and became more sporadic. This is the way your uterus progressively contracts back to its pre-pregnancy size.

I liked how I was with my baby the entire time. At a hospital, the mom and baby can be separated for up to a few hours after birth. At home, the midwife monitors the baby in the presence of the baby's parents or even in the arms of the mother or father. Having the baby and mom together is a priority when birthing at home. Any testing that can be done with the baby on the mother's arms is done this way.

My team also brought me a delicious soup to nourish me while they were checking the baby. I made sure to plan what I wanted that meal to be in advance. The first meal you eat after having your baby is very important. Your body has gone through a lot! The more nutritious that meal is the better. Keep in mind that nutrition is key for successful breastfeeding. JC bonded with our baby while I had my soup. It was a beautiful sight. And after I was done with my meal, we all rested on our comfortable bed and we took a nap.

Part Three: Comparing Your Options

Here are three tables to help you evaluate your options: Vaginal Birth vs. C-Section (**Table 11.3**), Baby's Health in a Vaginal Birth vs. C-Section (**Table 11.4**), and Home-Birth, Birthing Center, and Hospital Comparison (**Table 11.5**).

TABLE 11.3 VAGINAL BIRTH VS. C-SECTION

	Vaginal Birth		**C-Section**	
Cost	Home Birth $3,000-4,000 (approximately one-third of a hospital birth)[26]		Average $12,400[28]	
	Vaginal Hospital $10,445[27]		Hospital Services	
	Hospital Services		Fee:	$7,131
	Fee:	$5,517	Fee Details:	Price is for a 4-day admission. More days charged at $1,800 per day. Fewer days will reduce price by $1,800 per day.
	Fee Details:	Price is for a 2-day admission for mother and baby. More days charged at $1,800 per day for mother and $335 per day for baby.		
	Physician Services		Physician Services	
	Fee:	$4,086	Fee:	$4,517
	Fee Details:	Physician fee for procedure and routine postoperative care. Vaginal delivery of a baby	Fee Details:	Physician fee for procedure and routine postoperative care. Surgical delivery of a baby.
	Anesthesia		Anesthesia	
	Fee:	$842	Fee:	$750
	Fee Details:	Price is for an average surgery time of 2 hours. Prices may go up or down based upon the actual surgical time required.	Fee Details:	Price is for an average surgery time of 1 hour. Prices may go up or down based upon the actual surgical time required.

TABLE 11.3 CONT'D...

	Vaginal Birth	C-Section
Risk	Mortality risk to the delivering mother is far less severe than that of a C-section operation. Less interference from hospital staff means less emergency scenarios for mom and baby, giving both a higher rate of survival.[29]	Increases low-risk women's chances of certain rare, but potentially life-threatening problems, such as hemorrhage, blood clots, and bowel obstruction. More frequent risks include bladder damage, infection, and enduring pain.[30]
Future complications	Minimal risk.[31]	Greater likelihood of future complications in pregnancy, including uterine rupture or conditions in which the placenta covers the opening to the cervix (placenta previa), adheres abnormally to the uterine wall (placenta accreta), or separates from it (placenta abruption).[32]
Satisfaction of birth experience	Higher. Maternal satisfaction with vaginal delivery is high. Those who have experienced both modes of delivery would prefer vaginal birth on future pregnancies.[33]	Lower. Satisfaction with the birth experience is significantly lower among cesarean mothers and among those who had general anesthesia.[34]
Breastfeeding	Facilitates quicker, perhaps better, bonding with newborns. You can breastfeed right away. Breastfeeding prevalence in the delivery room is significantly higher after vaginal delivery compared with that after cesarean delivery.[35]	Baby may need to wait to nurse because of anesthesia. Mother may feel uncomfortable because of incision. The inability of women who have undergone a C-section to breastfeed comfortably in the delivery room and in the immediate postpartum period seems to be the explanation for them being less likely to breastfeed later on.[36]
Depression and post-traumatic stress	Reduced risk. Except in cases of Instrumental Vaginal Delivery.[37]	Greater risk than normal vaginal delivery, especially in cases of emergency C-section.[38]
Future pregnancies	No issues.	Longer-term impact. Higher risk for future ectopic pregnancies. Future fertility is lower than a woman who has a vaginal birth. More likely to experience serious problems with the placenta, like placenta previa, placenta accrete, or placental abruption.[39]

TABLE 11.4 BABY'S HEALTH IN A VAGINAL BIRTH VS. C-SECTION

	Vaginal Birth	C-Section
Risk	They may have trouble exiting the birth canal, such as when breech.	They may be cut or asphyxiate if the medical team has difficulty pulling them out.
Respiratory Issues	When your baby passes through your vaginal opening, the pressure helps to expel the amniotic fluid in your baby's lungs. This helps clear away any blockages in the lungs and nasal areas naturally rather than with extra medical attention.[40]	More likely to experience respiratory distress and have asthma later on.
Health	Coming through the birth canal prepares the baby for the outside world. Babies born vaginally receive a coating of immune-boosting microbes, and their intestines are more likely to have early colonization with beneficial bacteria—protections that babies delivered surgically miss out on.	Studies have found increased rates of obesity among American babies born by C-section. A bacterial deficit in babies' guts, some scientists speculate, may even be the factor that accounts for the higher obesity rates among them.
Breastfeeding Capacity	Easier.	Babies born via C-section may be somewhat drowsy and lethargic, especially if the mother was exposed to anesthetics for a prolonged period of time during labor.[41]
Future Babies	Normal.	The baby of a mother who has had one cesarean also seems to be at increased risk because it faces greater danger when growing in a uterus with a surgical scar.[42] The likelihood increases as the number of previous cesareans increases.[43]

TABLE 11.5 HOME-BIRTH, BIRTHING CENTER, AND HOSPITAL COMPARISON

	Home Birth	Birthing Center	Hospital
Interventions	Minimal	Minimal	High
Comfort	High. You have all of the comforts of your home available (own bed, bathtub, food, etc.). Complete privacy.	Medium. Homelike setting away from home. You go home the same day as birth. This may be pro or con. A car ride during contractions and then back home a few hours after giving birth may be uncomfortable.	Varies. You must travel to the hospital. The ambience is the least like home. Limited privacy, especially during delivery. Must stay overnight or longer for observation.
Freedom	High	Medium	Limited
Support	Midwives usually spend more time with laboring women than obstetricians do, and studies have shown that even passive, nonmedical support during labor leads to better birth outcomes. Midwives are more "invested" in vaginal deliveries by virtue of training and mindset. Because of this investment, they are more likely to help women give birth vaginally.		Nurses and doctors come in and out sporadically.
Safety	High. Your midwife is there to ensure your safety. You can trust her. A common perception is that women are safer with a doctor in a hospital, but studies show that both mothers and babies are safer with midwives. Births attended by Certified Nurse-Midwives (CNMs) produce fewer Cesarean sections, infant abrasions, complications, perineal lacerations, postpartum hemorrhage, and vacuum or forceps-assisted deliveries than physicians. Midwives can perform CPR or resuscitation and give Pitocin in the event of a potential hemorrhage.		Varies.

TABLE 11.5 CONT'D...

	Home Birth	Birthing Center	Hospital
Practitioner	Midwife. Although some physicians encourage midwifery, others adamantly oppose it. While OB/GYNs are specialists trained in interventions, which are sometimes necessary in complicated or high-risk pregnancies, midwives' training emphasizes skills that help women have healthy outcomes with as little intervention as possible. Popular pregnancy books will misinform you about midwives and their qualifications. Please note that midwives are experts at natural births. That is ALL they do, while OB/GYNs may mostly perform C-sections. Midwives are trained to do everything related to the care of a woman during pregnancy, except for C-sections/surgery.		OB/GYN or Certified Nurse Midwife
Cord Blood Care	Letting the cord pulsate all the blood and letting the placenta come out before cutting the umbilical cord is easy. No one is rushing you.	Same as home birth.	Time is limited and you may be rushed.
Stress	Birthing at home was comfortable and peaceful. No need to rush to the hospital. No need to pack your bags or load the car.	Medium. You need to get to the birthing center and check in. You then have to go home a few hours after the delivery.	Higher. You need to rush to the hospital, go through triage, etc.
Delivering the placenta	Delivers naturally.	Same as home birth.	Active management of third stage through fundal pressure.
Pulling the baby's neck	Midwives let the baby come naturally without pulling the neck. They may assist with the shoulders.	Same as home birth.	Happens frequently in a vaginal delivery and during a cesarean and it may injure the baby's neck.
Breastfeeding	Breastfeeding is better established at home where mom and baby stay together at all times. Keeping mom and baby together is important in the breastfeeding process. The sooner you can latch the baby to the mom, the easier it is going to be for that baby to breastfeed. Midwives are trained to help with breastfeeding.	You have the support of the staff in a home-like environment.	Lactation consultant available at hospital.

Action Step: Write your birth plan.

Who will deliver your baby? _____

Where will you deliver your baby? _____

Who is on your birthing team? _____

What interventions are you comfortable with? _____

What protocol is important to you? _____

_____

DELIVERING YOUR BABY

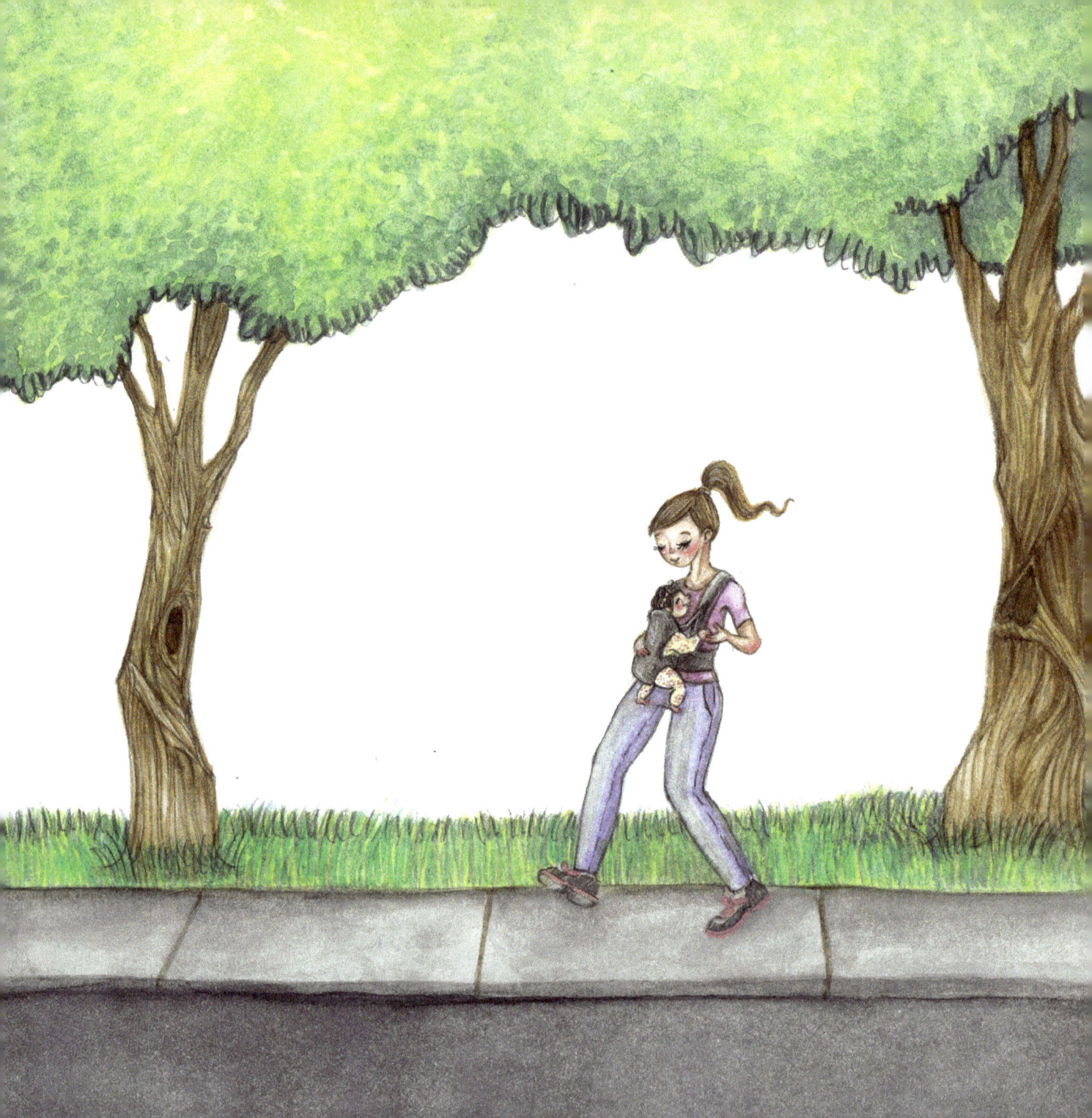

CHAPTER 12

Where Did My Body Go? Bouncing Back Post-Pregnancy

You may find that you still have a post-pregnancy belly after you deliver. This is normal. Your muscles stretched to accommodate your baby. Your uterus is still contracting for a few weeks until it gets back to its pre-pregnancy size. You may also be swollen and that can last for several days. Most women lose ten pounds immediately after they deliver. The baby weighs about seven pounds, and the placenta, blood, and amniotic fluid make up the other three pounds. The rest is the leftover pregnancy weight.

I really liked how Kate Middleton appeared in public after she delivered her baby looking like what a normal woman may look like after she delivers—still pregnant. Tom Sykes, *The Daily Beast's* royal correspondent, wrote, "This thoroughly modern royal was apparently determined to lend a helping hand to women everywhere who have just given birth, and shatter one of the last taboos of pregnancy—the post-baby belly."[1]

How I Bounced Back

Bella was only two days old when I weighed myself and realized that I had bounced back to my pre-pregnancy weight. I gained twenty pounds by week thirty-nine, but those extra pounds were gone just a few days after delivery. This was the result of following a healthy lifestyle before conception and during pregnancy.

I held on to fifteen pounds after Mila's birth. This may be because I was thinner and in great shape before getting pregnant with Mila. Fifteen pounds may not sound like much, but they were hard to get rid of. I began losing weight after making adjustments to my diet and starting a serious workout routine. Mila was six months old when I had five pounds to go, and it took me three months to shed those last five pounds. I achieved my pre-pregnancy weight by the time Mila was nine months old.

But I didn't stop there. I continued a workout program and a balanced diet after achieving my pre-pregnancy weight. Now Mila is one year old and I feel better than I have ever felt before. My self-confidence has increased and I have more energy to run after my children.

This is not about a quick fix. This is about bouncing back naturally and steadily so that your results last forever. Here is how I did it:

Immediately After You Deliver

Take time to rest. Your body has gone through a lot. Listen to your body. Do not push yourself during this stage. You don't want to get hurt. This will only complicate things for you and your family. So, tune in carefully.

Take care of your perineum. Women who have natural childbirths often feel great for a short while after delivering their babies. Natural birthing moms can get up shortly after labor and walk around or take a shower. However, there is the perineum. Hopefully you took care of it during pregnancy and massaged it to prevent tearing. You may feel sensitive in that area if you did experience tearing. Rinsing with an all-natural wash will help alleviate the stinging sensation when you use the bathroom. I like Feminine Fresh available at www.babybirthand-beyond.com. You can continue using the wash until the bleeding subsides. Mix three to four drops of the wash with lukewarm water in a peri-bottle. Then squirt the bottle on the area as you use the bathroom. The wash will neutralize the urine and reduce stinging. You can use it several times a day.

You can safely do some exercises in bed even immediately after you deliver if you feel like it. Kegels help your pelvic muscles, and

contracting your abs and buttocks at the same time begins strengthening your muscles.

Wear a girdle. Put on a corset or girdle as soon as you feel up for it. Wear it as fast as possible and as much as possible for up to twelve months. It will feel tight and uncomfortable, but it will bring back your hourglass shape—guaranteed! I used an Ann Chery Colombian girdle.

Choose to breastfeed. Breastfeeding not only helps your uterus contract faster, which helps reduce abdominal swelling, but it is also a natural way of shedding those extra pounds. A year of breastfeeding, with proper nutrition and an active lifestyle may result in a hotter body than before. (Read Chapter 10 for the endless benefits of breastfeeding.)

Watch what you eat. First of all, your body has been through a lot. Imagine you just ran a marathon. You need to replenish your body with nutrients and vitamins. This is especially true if you are breastfeeding because your body draws nutrients from your blood to produce nourishing breast milk. Eat healthy fats, proteins, and vegetables. Stay away from empty calories and starches that will only cause additional bloating.

Get checked by a chiropractor. The process of giving birth may cause subluxations in your spine that can later result in back pain or other health issues. The sooner you fix it, the better.

As Soon As You Feel Up For It

Remember it is important to tune in to your body! You can start doing the following whenever you feel ready.

Prevent postpartum depression. You may have heard of postpartum depression or the baby blues. My naturopath explained to me that it takes one year for hormones to stabilize postpartum, but that diet and exercise help accelerate the process. You can also try supplementing with these great foods:

> Maca root has long been recognized as an energy enhancer and mood stabilizer. It has traditionally been used to treat PMS and menopause. It's nutritious and powerfully complex, with life-giving and beauty-enhancing ingredients such as phytonutrients, amino acids, vitamins, and fatty acids. I added a tablespoon to my smoothie in the mornings.

> Take fish oil supplements. I like Carlson's Fish Oil. They are a solid company and their oils come from low-mercury fish. You can begin taking these during pregnancy. Studies show that fish oils help prevent postpartum depression.[2] Fish oil also helps treat

acne, which can sometimes surface after pregnancy due to stabilizing hormones.

Go for a daily walk postpartum. Walking is not only good for your body and mind, but it's also beneficial for your baby. Newborns need vitamin D, and the sun offers it in its most natural form. You can begin walking around your neighborhood as soon as you feel up for it; just remember to take it easy. You can also use a baby carrier if your baby gets fussy in the stroller. I have the organic Ergo baby carrier.

Keep tabs on your weight. Weigh yourself at home, on the same scale, at least once a week. But don't do this if it stresses you out. Stress actually causes some people to overeat and then gain weight.

Establish a goal. Figure out how much you want to lose, by when, and how you plan on accomplishing that.

Recruit an accountability partner. Share your goal with a person you can trust and ask him or her to keep you accountable.

Treat any stretch marks. Fitness Magazine says that the key to eliminating stretch marks is to treat them early. There are powerful home remedies that you can start applying on the stretch marks whenever you are ready, such as olive oil, lemon juice, and aloe.

Visit a naturopath. I felt like those extra pounds were never going to leave after three months. I accepted the fact that it was just going to take longer. I visited my naturopath, and she told me it was better to tackle those pounds early on because it would take me longer to bounce back if I let them linger. I tried blaming it on my age or the fact that this was my second pregnancy, but she didn't buy it. She quickly noticed that my diet was loaded with carbs when she asked me about my eating habits. I wish I had gone to her sooner because I saw results right away as soon as I changed my diet. I lost seven pounds the following month.

At Six Weeks and Beyond.

Get a haircut. "Up to 50% of women experience an increased shedding period after giving birth. 'It's called telogen effluvium, and it occurs anywhere from one to six months after giving birth,' says Francesca Fusco, MD, assistant clinical professor of dermatology at Mount Sinai School of Medicine in New York City."[3] Getting a cut will make you look and feel better. Bonus points if you can sneak in a manicure and pedicure. It's nice for new moms to treat themselves every once in a while.

Implement a workout routine. Your healthcare practitioner may tell you to wait six weeks before exercising. Start with caution and build up slowly. I started an aerobics program at six weeks and modified difficult movements to avoid getting hurt.

Join a workout group. I began a running routine when Mila was two months old. I knew the cardio was beneficial for my heart, overall health, and would help me burn the extra calories. I found that running was very relaxing and helped me think. It was beneficial for my body, mind, and soul. I eventually joined a running group about six months after Mila was born and this increased my consistency.

Post about your bounce back process if you are active on social media. You may be encouraged by the support of others and enjoy the comments on your journey to bounce back.

Work on your abs. I joined a CrossFit garage to work on toning my body. My CrossFit coach says that abs are made in the kitchen. Cutting empty carbs and sugar will reduce bloating and any extra fat that may be lingering in the tummy area. Cardio and core exercises will also help you get your abs back. All these exercises help strengthen your core:

- Planking for as long as you can hold it and then releasing
- Burpees
- Sit ups with double padding for your lower back and buttocks
- Push-ups

Hydrate and replenish. Your skin has stretched in many places. Make sure to drink at least eight glasses of water per day to help bring it back. Drink more if you are breastfeeding. Collagen also helps with skin elasticity. You can take citric juices and vitamin C to increase collagen production.

Visit your health practitioner. Getting a check-up will ensure you identify and take care of any issues. Getting blood work done before you go to your practitioner will make your visit more productive, so make sure to ask for a lab order when you make your appointment.

You can do it! We are really hard on ourselves sometimes. We want to bounce back to the way we looked before getting pregnant, but we doubt our ability to do so. I want you to know that you can do it!

There are days when you may feel tired. But remember that this program is for you when you are struggling. It is not for anyone else. These activities benefit you, your health, your stamina, and your self-confidence. Bouncing back is an investment in YOURSELF.

It will be much easier for you to bounce back if you do what I've laid out in this book throughout your pregnancy and afterwards. It surely helped me. However, I wasn't always like this. As I have shared with you, there was a time in my late teens when I suffered from severe asthma. I couldn't even walk long distances without getting an asthma attack. This is why my achievements in sports are nothing short of a miracle. My first goal when I started running was to run a 5K (3.1 miles). I am now running 7 miles in 80 minutes and my new goal is to run a half marathon.

The best results are the ones you achieve through steady work and commitment. Bouncing back is not easy, but it's also not impossible. It's not going to be harder than labor or breastfeeding—that's for sure. I know you will be able to achieve your goal, and I'd love to hear about it when you do!

Action Step: Write your Bouncing Back Plan. The simple version of mine was easy to remember. 1) Get in shape. 2) Get a tan. 3) Get a new wardrobe. I made sure to tell many friends who would keep me accountable. What's yours?

_____

_____

_____

_____

_____

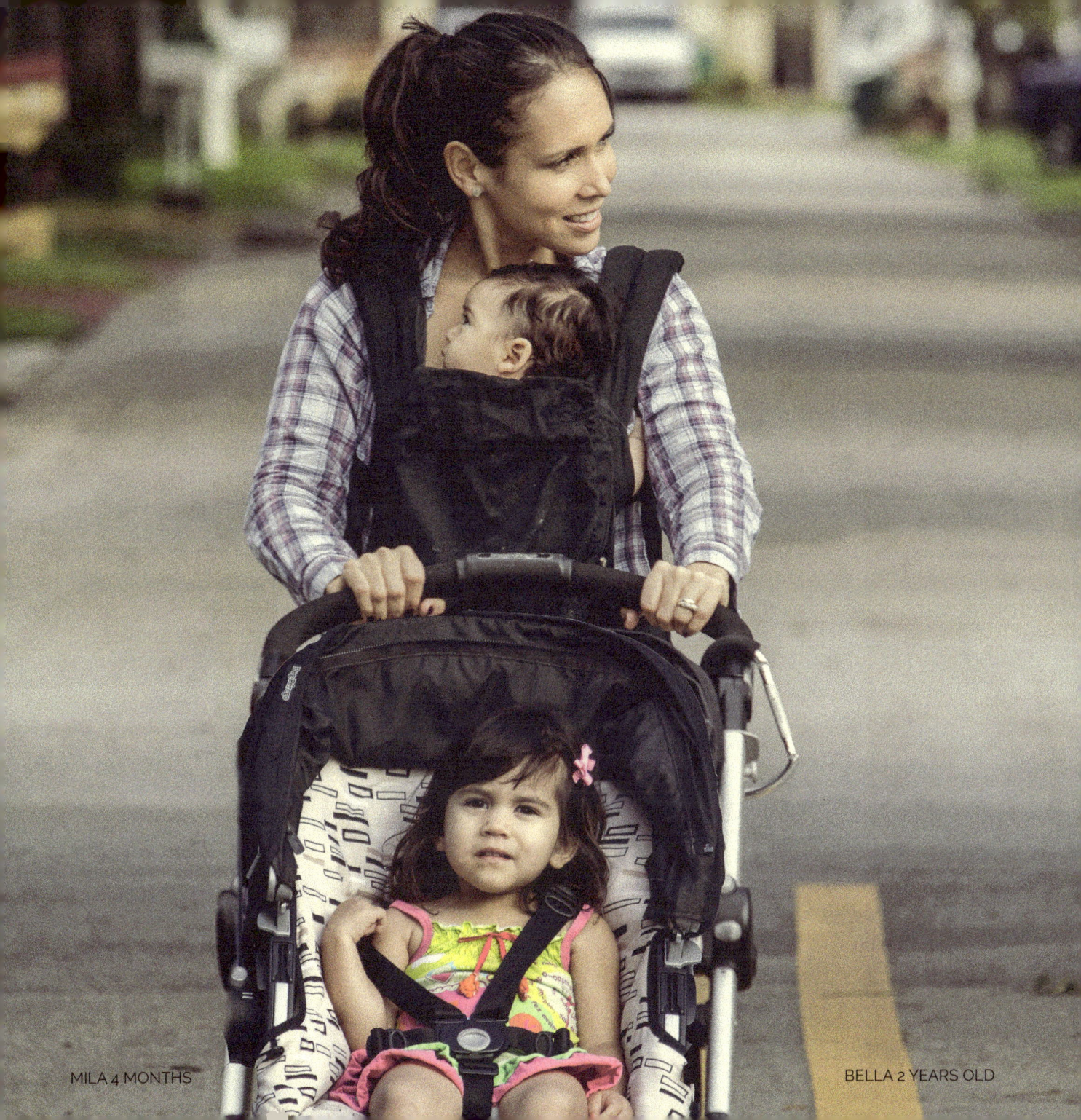

MILA 4 MONTHS

BELLA 2 YEARS OLD

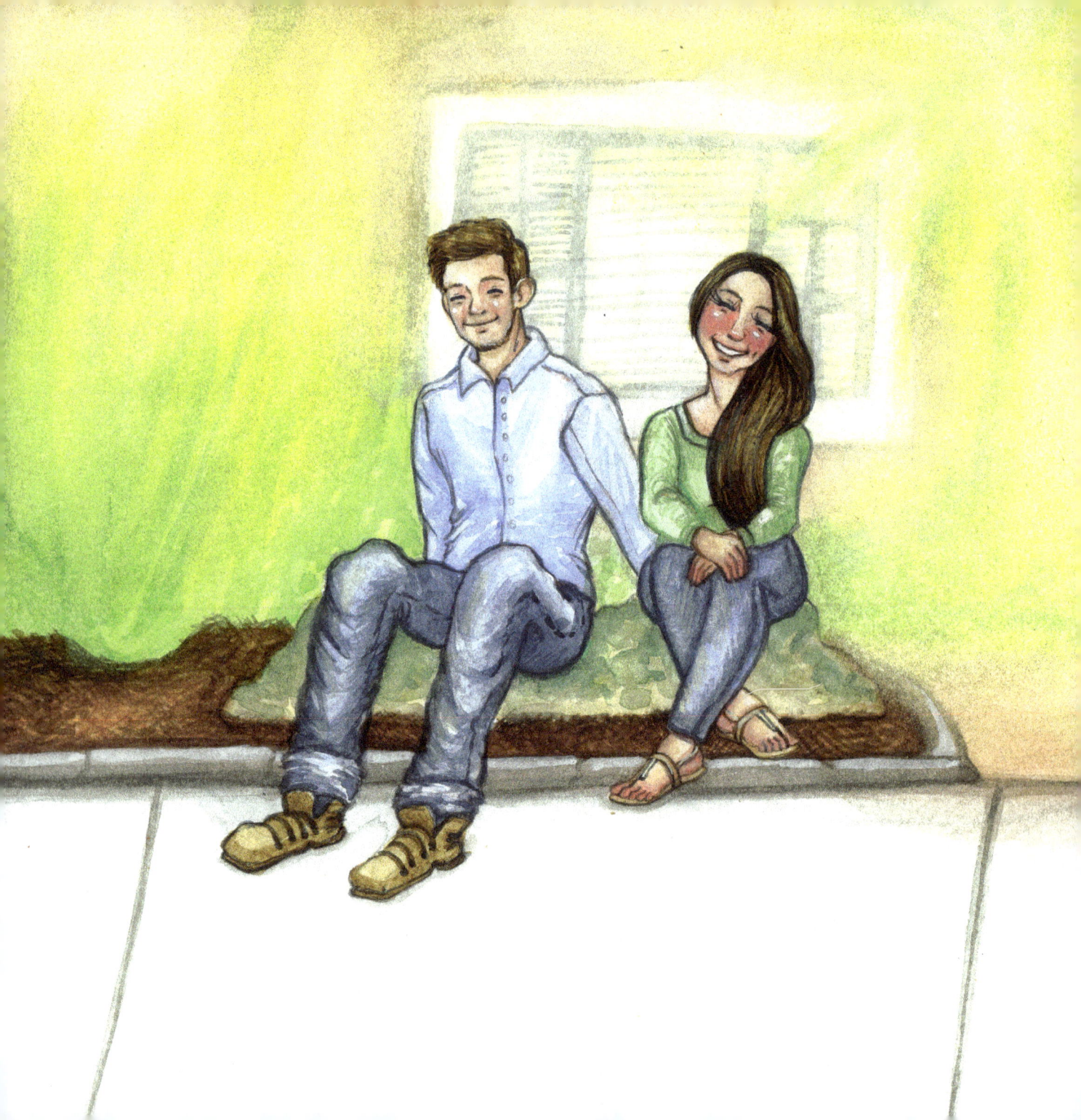

CHAPTER 13

Pain-Free Delivery

I have been a youth leader at my church and other organizations ever since I turned 18. My husband and I quickly decided to serve in the youth ministry when we moved to Miami and found a church to attend. My life began taking unexpected turns in June of 2009. That's when I met my older kids—Abi and John.

I have always felt a deep desire to share our adoption story. I will tell you how I became a mom of two teenagers at a very young age. Some may argue that adoption doesn't really fit in a pregnancy book, but I think that you will appreciate learning about it because it's part of my journey to *motherhood*.

I consider myself lucky to have been a Christian from a very young age. My mom and I went to church every single Sunday ever since I was a child. My parents divorced when I was very young, but I had the blessing of having my grandparents around while growing up. They taught me so much. They, along with my mom, truly believed I could be anything I wanted to be. And they always made sure I knew that.

I had just finished my bachelor's degree in business at the University of Puerto Rico. I did very well, finished in three years, and even graduated with honors. My next step was to either get a job or start my graduate degree immediately. I was already admitted into my school's graduate program. I didn't know what to do, and I knew my choice would impact the rest of my life. I wrote a letter to God asking Him for guidance. I explained that I needed his help—I needed to know which way to go. I received a call from a Fortune 500 medical devices company in Miami Lakes, Florida less than one week later. The opportunity was my dream job. I quickly went through the interview process and got the job. There was no doubt in my mind that God had answered my letter.

I left for Miami with a one-way ticket. My mom came with me to help me relocate. That Sunday, we saw a sign for a church while walking around my new neighborhood. We checked it out the following weekend, and Calvary Fellowship has been my home church ever since.

I started the job and quickly got the hang of it. The company was pleased with my work, and they began paying for my master's degree at the University of Miami one year later. I finished my master's with academic excellence. After that, my company sent me to Harvard University for an Executive Leadership Program. I was promoted to different positions every eighteen months, eventually becoming the head of human resources for the Latin America division.

JC was also doing great. He earned a scholarship for law school and ranked first among his graduating class. He landed a great job as an Associate Attorney at a growing law firm.

We went from a small apartment to a big house and from sharing one used car to having two new cars. We were young, happy, and successful. But one day, my grandfather passed away unexpectedly. I always worried about my grandmother because she was the one who was sick with Alzheimer's. I never thought that he would be the first to leave. His death really affected me and I held on to my faith for strength. I felt so broken while at church one Sunday morning. I remember we were singing *Hosanna* by Hillsong. There is a part of the song that says, "Break my heart for what breaks yours. Everything I am for your Kingdom's cause."[1] I joined in the singing with great conviction and prayed that God would really take every part of me, like the song said.

Things at work started getting tough soon after. I felt like they didn't want me there anymore, and I was unhappy. I told my boss I was going to start looking for another job—in the middle of an economic crisis. This was in May 2009—when people were doing their best to hold on to their jobs instead of quitting! God is so faithful that I was offered a job at my church before my last official day at my old job.

It turns out that they *always* wanted to hire me but never thought I would leave my old job. Our

THE SECRETS TO A HEALTHY PREGNANCY

Youth Pastor invited me to attend a chapel service at a local orphanage during my first week working at the church. That is where I met Abi and John and their half-brother Guillermo.

I felt a connection as soon as I met them. God placed them in my heart, and I felt a big burden to be their mom. I was never interested in adopting, but the love I felt for them—almost immediately—was out of this world.

I will never forget how they were sitting side by side and almost looked like twins, even though Abi was sixteen and John was fourteen. They both looked so sad.

I went up to them just like I did with some of the other kids there. I talked to them for a bit and tried to make them smile. I asked one of the staff members about them when they left. He told me they had a half-brother that was three-and-a-half years old and that a family in North Carolina was going to adopt them. Hearing about their adoption made me feel strange. I should have been happy for them, but I felt weird—almost as if I was the one meant to be their mother.

I kept going to the orphanage every week and helped during chapel time in preparation for a summer camp that our church was planning. I enjoyed serving all of the kids there, but I especially loved seeing Abi and John. I felt such a big connection that one afternoon, after chapel, I called the administrative office and asked about them once again. This time they told me that a friend of their biological mom was going to adopt them. They told me that she picked them up every weekend. I thought, "Okay, that's that."

I saw Abi sitting next to a boy when I returned for chapel the following week. I saw his hand on her leg and immediately felt very protective over her. I wanted to make sure she would be okay, so after the chapel I talked to her about boys and we basically had the sex talk, and we connected. I asked her about how she ended up there, and she shared her story with me. She told me they were taken away from their mom because of their mother's addiction only about a month earlier. I asked her what was going to happen to them, and she told me she wanted to age out of the foster system and get custody of her younger siblings, John and Guillermo.

I was surprised to hear that she wanted to do this. I never thought she would be so brave. I asked her if she would ever want to be adopted or fostered, and she said she didn't. I remember hugging her and crying with her.

That day, I went back home and prayed for them. We had two empty rooms in our house: the guest room, which had a queen size bed, and the game room. I thought, "How could those kids be in an orphanage when we have two spare rooms at home?" I felt that Abi could have the guest room, and the boys could have the playroom. We even had two twin beds in our garage from our guest room back at our old apartment. We had everything we needed to accommodate them.

That weekend, JC and I were walking our dogs to the coffee shop and I asked him if he thought it would be crazy to adopt three kids from this orphanage. He said, "Yes." We both laughed and I began sharing with him about the kids. I told him he had to meet them. I wondered if this was something we had to do.

JC and I planned on going to Europe and begin trying to conceive around this time. We had two plane tickets to Paris and were leaving on JC's birthday. Adopting wasn't even remotely in our plans.

JC didn't feel right about it at that moment. He didn't even know them, and I didn't even know much about them. What if something went wrong? Still, I felt very strongly about JC meeting them, so I prayed about it.

JC was finally able to make it to the chapel service the week before the summer camp. I was so nervous about them meeting, because I knew I would finally get my answer. I introduced JC to both of them. Then, after chapel, JC (an introvert) went to John and the other young boys to try and make some conversation. He asked them if they liked playing sports. The kids started talking about basketball and American football. My husband is a soccer fan—he played soccer since he was a young kid all the way through college. So, he asked if any of them liked soccer. The kids started saying, "Nah! We don't like soccer." But after they quieted down, my son John (another introvert) spoke up and said, "I like soccer." That was it. That was all he said. And that was the spark that started their relationship. I asked JC what he thought after the chapel service was over and he smiled at me and nodded yes. I couldn't believe it!

The summer camp was the following week. As a counselor, I had the responsibility of bringing dinner to one of the houses at the orphanage for the entire week. I made sure that I was assigned to their house so I could get to know them better and vice versa. JC had a very busy schedule with work, but he made time to join us for dinner. We enjoyed connecting with their half-brother Guillermo during dinnertime, even though he was in time-out for most of the time.

We had a great time during camp. We poured our love on them. We cried and laughed with them. The last day of camp was hard. We had to say goodbye and I could tell it was hard for them too. I gave them each something to remember me by when I said bye to them. I also

158   THE SECRETS TO A HEALTHY PREGNANCY

promised Abi I would continue to visit them every week.

John got permission to go play soccer with JC the Saturday after camp ended. They also attended our church for the first time that Sunday. The staff at the orphanage got to know us little by little, and they started allowing us to have events at our house for the kids. We spent a lot of time together with Abi, John, and some of the other kids, having movie nights and just hanging out.

Weeks passed and they got to know us, our home, and our extended family. They knew that we cared for them, but they didn't know the extent of our love. They didn't know we wanted to adopt them. We waited until we had no doubt that we wanted them to be our kids and until we felt they knew us well enough to know if they wanted us to be in their lives more permanently. The day we decided to talk to them about becoming more to them was very special. We planned what we were going to say and when to say it. Almost like a proposal. We went to see them at the orphanage that night and took board games and pizza. We asked if we could speak with both of them outside before leaving.

JC did most of the talking, just like we planned. I also spoke to them from my heart. We told them we loved them and Guillermo, and we wanted to be there for them as much as they wanted us to be. We could be their friends (like we already were), but we could also be more. From mentors, to foster parents, or even adoptive parents—"Everything!" I will never forget the look on their faces the day we proposed to them—their teary big blue eyes in awe of what we were saying. We told them we didn't want them to give us an answer yet. We wanted them to think about it and discuss it among themselves on their own and to let us know another day.

They went to church with us the following day, and we went to the mall afterwards. I remember we were in the food court when they told us they wanted to talk to us. We all sat around a table, and they told us they had thought about what we had told them the previous night and that they wanted "everything!" We were so happy. JC and I asked them if they were sure, if they needed more time to think. But we all wanted the same thing. We wanted to be a family!

We had a lot of support in making the adoption process as fast as possible because they were already in foster care. They moved in with us on JC's birthday—the exact same day we were supposed to leave to Paris. We also wanted to adopt Guillermo, but the court granted his biological father full custody after six months. We still see him every once in a while and on special occasions. Abi and John are in college. Abi wants to become a social worker, and John is studying business with plans of attending law school.

I always wanted to be a young mom. I thought that I would have my first baby at 27, just like my mom did. It turns out that I had three kids at twenty-seven, and two of them were already taller than me! Parenting teenagers isn't easy. But maybe we were made parents for a time like this, just like Esther from the Bible was made queen to rescue her people. We trained all of our lives for this—growing up in a Christian home and spending years working with the youth.

It's scary to think that I would have never met my older kids if I hadn't left that company. My life could have turned out so differently. This book may not even exist. Even as a Christian, I was missing out on God's blessings until the day I decided to surrender it all to Him—to let go of my own desires. That day, I decided to trust God no matter the outcome. And oh, what a precious gift He gave me: *the gift of motherhood*.

Action Step: Volunteer at your local children's home.

My local children's home is: _____

Address: _____

Phone number: _____

Dates when I'm available to serve on: _____

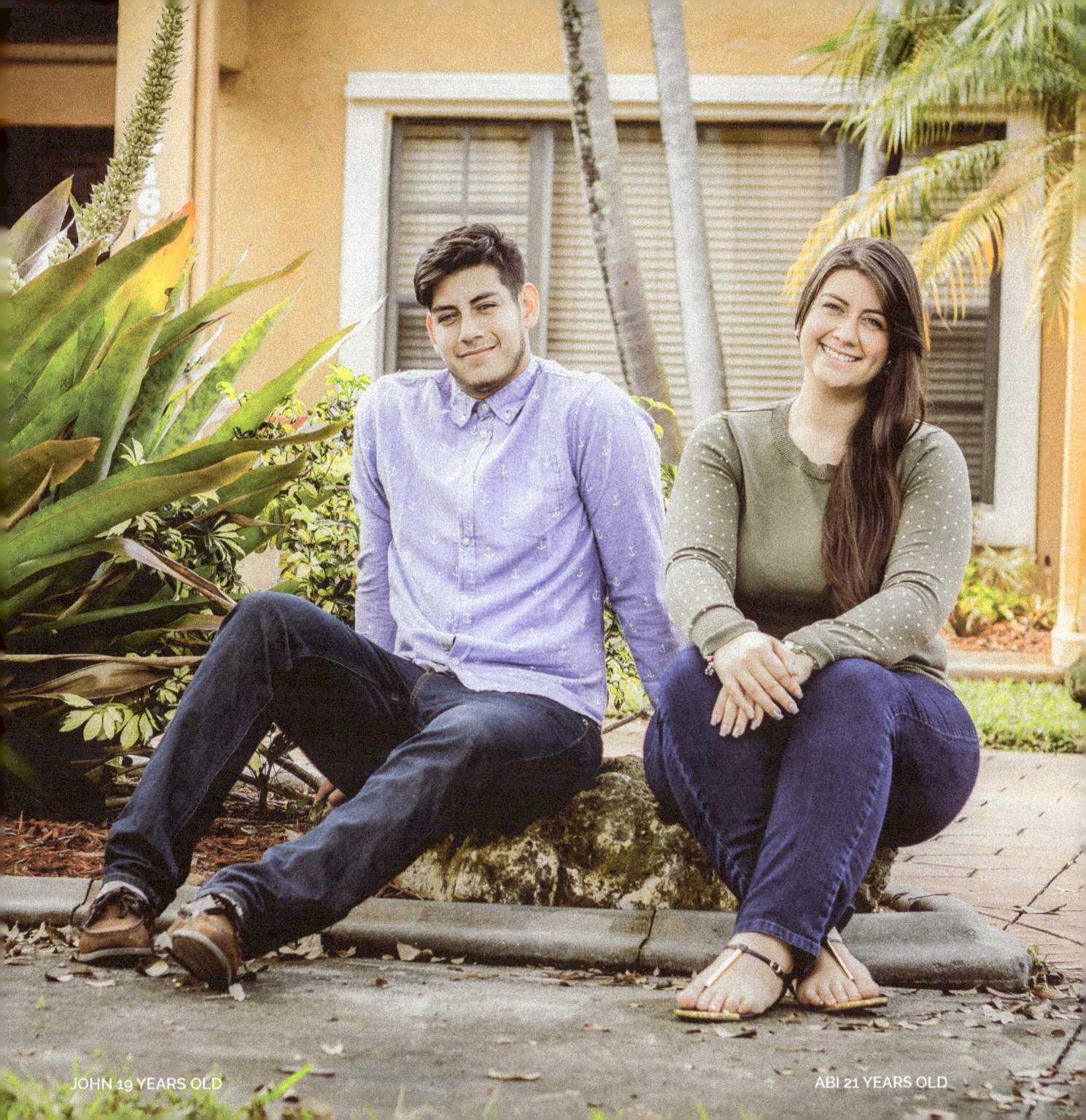

JOHN 19 YEARS OLD

ABI 21 YEARS OLD

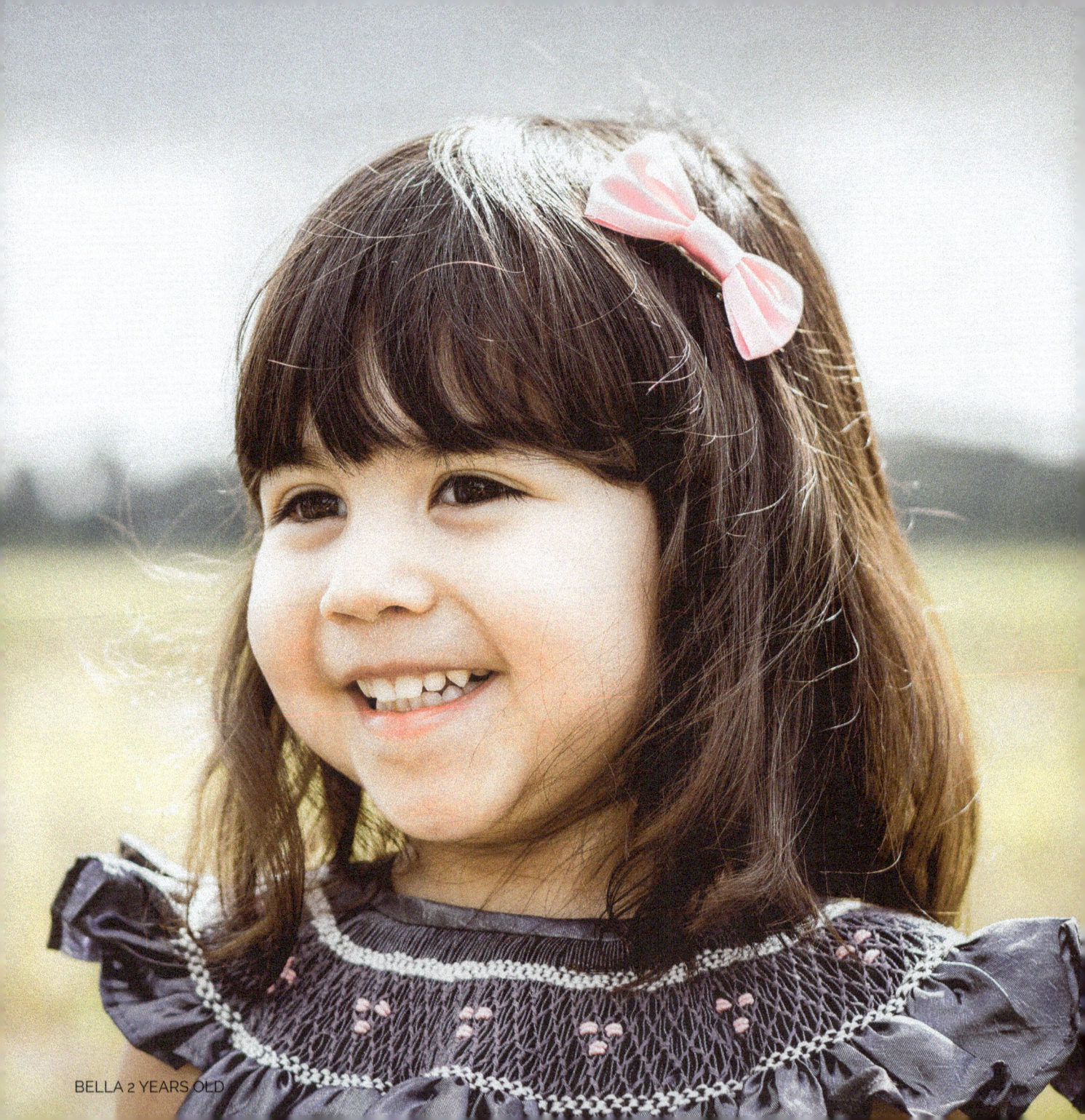

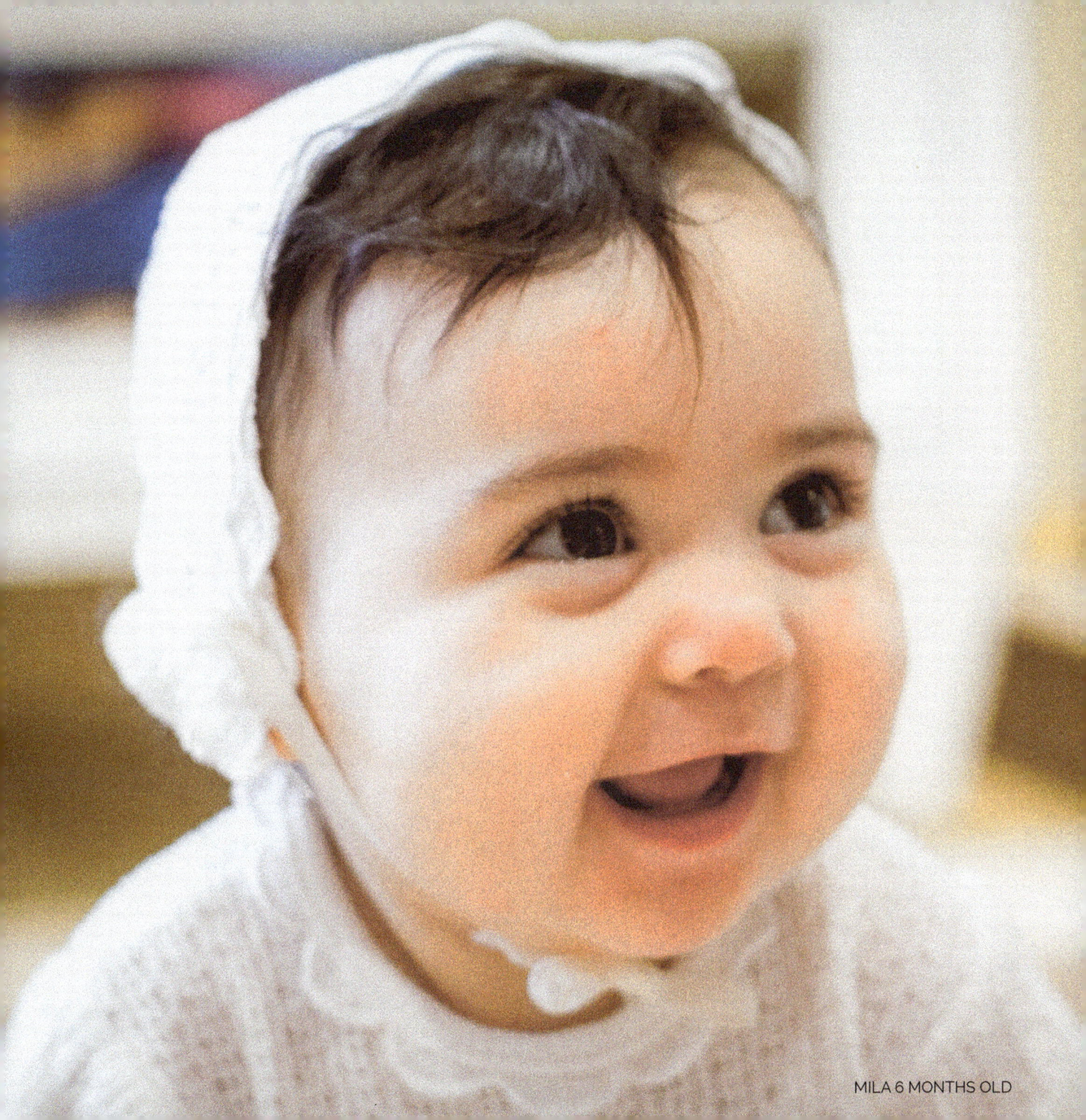

MILA 6 MONTHS OLD

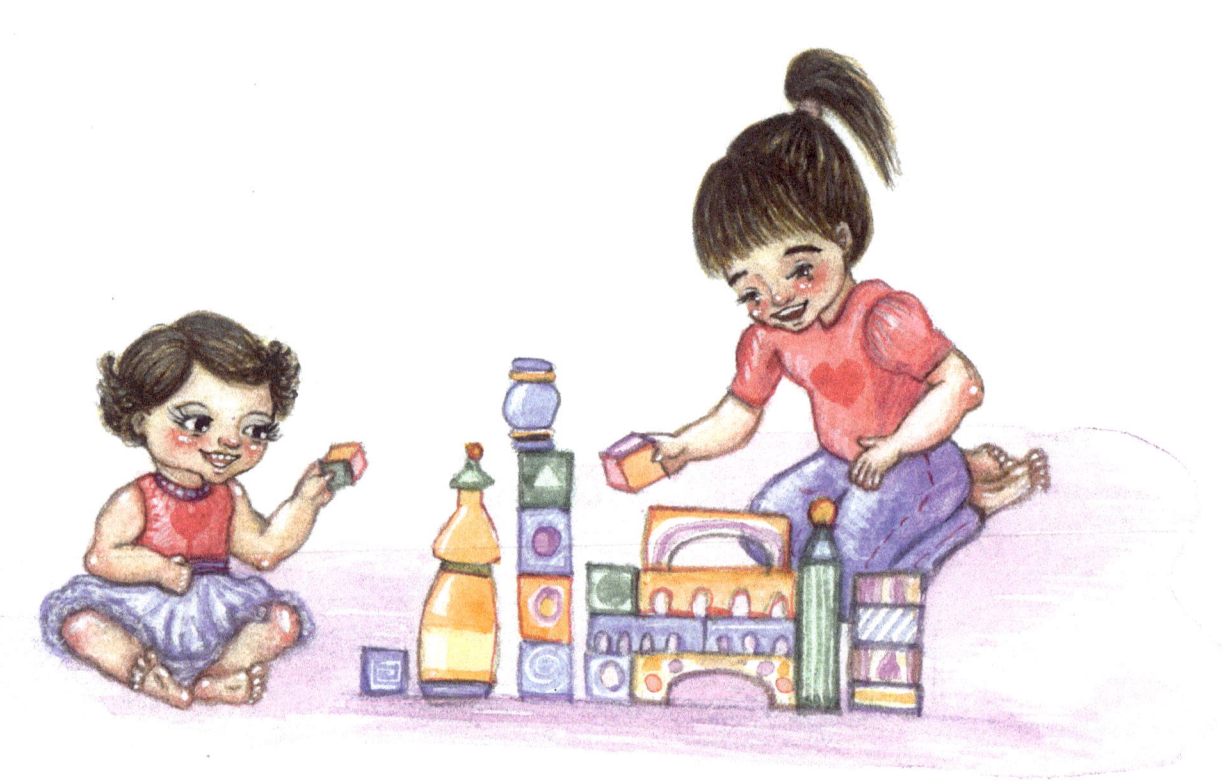

BONUS CHAPTER

Healthy Babies

I was presenting at a conference in Coral Gables and received a call from my friend Ana who was taking care of Bella. I took the call and immediately realized that something was wrong. Ana was panicking as she screamed that Bella, my two-year old, was having a seizure. It took me a second to tell her to call 911. I hung up, apologized to my clients, and told them I had to leave.

I cannot describe the terror and desperation I felt as I left that conference room. I was angry with myself for being away from home. My daughter needed me, and I needed to be with her. I realized that one of the clients, Cristina, was following me as I ran down the hotel stairs to the lobby. She must have seen how anxious I was because she asked if I wanted her to come with me when I got to my car. I said yes, even though I barely knew her, because I felt she would be helpful.

I am so glad Cristina came with me because I freak out after ten minutes of driving through busy streets and violating transit regulations. I freaked out when I realized I had been driving around in circles the entire time. Cristina was busy trying to call the different numbers that I gave her to reach JC, so she hadn't noticed either. I started yelling at myself and couldn't believe I wasted all that time. She told me to calm down and to let her drive. That's the moment when I felt she became my angel as she drove me home safely.

I called everyone who I thought needed to go to my house while Cristina drove, including Dr. Lisa, our chiropractor. I was so frustrated by the traffic and the fact that I wasn't home. I remember crying, but being so stressed that the tears wouldn't come out. I just wished that I could hold Bella at that very moment.

This had never happened before. Bella was a healthy baby. I immediately knew this was caused by a fever. She woke up with a swollen eye two days earlier. We went to our chiropractic appointment, and her eye was better that same afternoon. She woke up with a mild fever the next day, so JC and I decided to keep her with us during the church service, instead of taking her to Sunday school. Bella was fine that afternoon.

I had plans to take Bella to the chiropractor that Monday morning. I knew that an adjustment would help her body fight whatever was causing the fever. However, I overslept and didn't think I had enough time to take her and be back on time for my presentation later that day. I was rushing to leave when Ana arrived, and I barely explained to her that Bella was fighting something. It never crossed my mind to make sure she was drinking enough water. So many regrets crossed my mind while Cristina drove me home that afternoon.

I kept making phone calls on the way home to avoid regretting everything and thinking about the things I wish I had done. I talked to the paramedic who arrived at the house, and he confirmed that Bella experienced a febrile seizure. He told me that she was okay and to treat and monitor her fever. The paramedics were gone by the time I got home, but JC was already there with Bella. I immediately held her and checked to see how she was doing. She looked very tired, but otherwise okay. I hugged so her hard. Then, I hugged JC while still holding Bella.

I spoke to Dr. Lisa who rushed out of her practice to check Bella and adjust her. She told me Bella was fine and to make sure I kept her hydrated.

Bella kept fighting the illness for the next few days. Her fevers ranged from 100-104°F. I kept treating her naturally and praying for her. One night, I was worried about her and begged God to heal her. The fever was gone the following day and never came back. I learned so many things about infant immune systems and natural treatments during that stressful week.

Bella is now three years old, and being her mom has taught me so much about how to keep a baby healthy. Mila just turned one, and she is a very healthy baby just like her sister. Looking back, I know that Ana was the best person who

could have been with Bella during her seizure. Ana's son, Gabriel, and two of her other children suffer from epilepsy. She knew exactly what to do, and God only knows how I would have reacted in that situation.

Ana has learned so much about alternative medicine since that day. Gabriel had a serious epilepsy attack one month after Bella's seizure. He suffered from over a dozen seizures in one day. He had been to the best doctors after he was diagnosed with epilepsy at only sixteen months old, but he was not getting any better. Gabriel was now twenty-seven years old, and the doctors kept increasing his dosage for an array of medications. His quality of life was decreasing; it was hard for him to wake up in the morning and he was very slow to react.

Gabriel had a seizure three months earlier, which caused him to crash his car into a building's metal fence. His car was almost a total loss, but thankfully he was okay and nobody else was hurt. Ana was scared after these two episodes happened so close to each other. My mom and I had been telling her about chiropractic and alternative medicine. After this last episode, my mom was convinced that they couldn't wait any longer and drove them to our naturopath in hopes of finding something different to help Gabriel.

Gabriel began getting treatment with my naturopath and my chiropractor on the same week. His change was almost immediate. He had more energy and was more alert within one week. He hasn't had another seizure to this day. Gabriel looks happier and healthier than ever before. We continue to pray for Gabriel and have faith that he is healed.

It broke my heart to hear Ana say that she wished someone told her about these other options while Gabriel was younger. She explained to me that she went to many doctors—even to the best neurologist in the city—and they all told her he had a genetic disorder, and all they could do was increase his medications. She wonders why none of them told her that something else was out there. Perhaps Gabriel could have been a healthy child. Maybe he could have had an easier life. But they just didn't know. That's why I am sharing this with you. Knowledge is power. You have the power to affect your lives and the lives of those around you.

The objective of this chapter is to establish a foundation for the care of your baby and other children. Even healthy babies get sick. But there are healthy alternatives for fighting illnesses and different ways to treat them that will help your baby be stronger going forward. Here are my ten commandments for healthy babies to help you get started.

The Ten Commandments For Raising Healthy Babies

Have a happy home. Stress affects children just like it affects adults in the three following areas: physically, mentally, and emotionally. A happy home begins with love, communication, and respect for all members of the family. Listen to your baby's cues and let your children know that you understand what they are telling you. Lead by example by communicating how you are feeling, your plans, etc. For example, I tell my toddler when I am tired so that she knows how I feel, and she isn't surprised by my atypical behavior. When my baby is crying, I listen to her cry and try to understand what it is she wants. I want them to learn early on that what they say is important to me. This way, they feel encouraged to communicate with me in the future.

Our homes can become hectic at times. The key is avoiding those moments. You can prevent stress by planning ahead by having routines so that your child knows how to behave, and disciplining your child. Yes, this is a way to reduce stress, especially in the long run. We do time-outs for our toddler. She first gets a clear warning then goes to time-out if she still does not conform. Being consistent in disciplining helps your child behave better and makes you a happier parent. A happier parent leads to a happier home, which leads to happier babies.

Ensure good nutrition. Watch what they eat and drink. Breast milk is the best food for at least the first six months. Follow your baby's cues in determining if he or she is ready to start eating solids. It's fun to feed your child different foods, but be careful not to do it too soon. You may find that it causes your baby to lose interest in nursing and reject the breast sooner than you wished. The Weston Price Foundation has a great timeline to follow when starting first foods. This website also contains a great recipe to make formula using goat's milk. Try to buy organic produce. The amount of pesticides in conventional produce affects your children's small bodies more than ours because their internal organs are still developing and maturing.[1]

Make sure your baby exercises. Exercise is very beneficial in developing your baby's motor skills and overall health. I find that my girls are calmer, nap easier, and sleep better at night after they exercise. Remember that you are also forming habits. Now is the time to start if you want a healthy and active teenager. "Infancy and the toddler years are the time that the brain is developing pathways and connections to the muscles. Children who do not get enough exercise may miss out on the chance to make the strong kinds of brain-muscle connections that make physical activity easier and more enjoyable."[2] My two young girls started

swimming lessons before they could even walk. Swimming is a great exercise and important in preventing devastating accidents.

Make sure your baby has enough down time. Rest is even more important for babies and children than it is for adults—especially when they are fighting an illness. Their bodies are growing quickly, and rest is a time to rebuild energy during times of growth spurts. Implementing a napping schedule is one of the best things you can do for their physical, mental, and emotional health. An overtired child will be more irritable, less alert, and more susceptible to illnesses than a rested child.

Make your baby's health a priority. I was so worried about making sure I had all the materials ready for my big day on the day Bella had a seizure, that I put those things before her needs. She was sick, and I didn't even notice because I was distracted with everything else. Learn from my mistake and don't let it happen to you.

Learn about your baby's health. Dedicate time to researching how your child's immune system works and ways you can aid in his or her mental and emotional development. The Internet has made it easy to do endless amounts of research, so don't just trust one source. Evaluate things like when to begin exposing your kids to television. After you feel you have researched long enough, trust your instincts and make a well-reasoned decision that you are comfortable with.

Prevent illnesses. Nutritional supplements like Vitamin D drops for exclusively breast-fed babies and Cod Liver Oil are very beneficial in building a baby's immune system. I give my girls Carlson's Cod Liver Oil in bubble gum flavor once a day. Bella also takes Jarrow Formulas Yum-Yum Dophilus probiotics. Your kids will almost inevitably get sick, especially when they are around many other children. I believe this is part of these early years. Looking back, however, I did notice that Bella began getting sick when I stopped giving her a daily dose of cod liver oil. There was a time when I took Bella to work with me, and my boss would ask me why she smelled like fish. I felt bad for my little baby and gradually stopped giving it to her. I have noticed the huge difference it makes in her ability to fight a cold and recover now that she is taking it again. I have also learned tricks to prevent the fishy scent, like giving the cod liver oil before bath time so that spills don't liger on their bodies or clothes.

Avoid unnecessary antibiotics and vaccines. The problem with antibiotics is that your body gets used to depending on them to fight off bacteria instead of building its immune system to fight it. The body can build immunity against antibiotics in cases of overuse. In addition, antibiotics kill both the bad and good bacteria. Good bacteria are vital for proper digestive system function, which is fundamental for a strong immune system. "The good bacteria tell your body how much nutrition they need, and your body responds by supplying just that much and no more—so that any excess bad bacteria are starved out. The helpful bacteria also produce a substance that kills harmful microbes."[3] So, instead of giving your baby too many antibiotics, you can give probiotics, which will increase the volume of good bacteria.

Vaccines are a controversial topic. My naturopath doesn't recommend using vaccinations to help immunity. She says she never vaccinated her three children who are now healthy adults. They all did sports without any disease and have traveled the world. She explains, "Vaccines are a risk. You don't know what they can put in the vaccine. The child's immune system can have an adverse effect. I will not run the risk." I was shocked to learn that vaccines have been recalled due to dangers caused to children and that they could even contain aborted fetus. There are websites that contain information that is crucial for you to learn before vaccinating your child, such as *www.Vacinfo.org*, *www.nvic.org*, and *www.whale.to/vaccines.html*.

Choose your pediatrician carefully. Your child's pediatrician or healthcare practitioner can be a great resource and guidance during times of uncertainty. It is very important for you pick one that is congruent with your health belief system. There are many pediatricians who favor using alternative medicine and minimizing interventions. I have a pediatrician that is very supportive of breastfeeding and intervening only when necessary. He is also understanding of my stance on vaccines. However, our family doctor is our chiropractor, Dr. Lisa. I make sure to take my girls to the chiropractor whenever they get sick so they can get checked and corrected if necessary.

I also sought the help of an Acupuncture Physician (AP) during a time when Bella was getting frequent colds. An AP is a great alternative for curing allergies and asthma. She tested Bella for allergies and treated her with a non-invasive technique called NAET that same day. NAET uses a blend of selective energy balancing, testing and treatment procedures from acupuncture/acupressure, allopathy, chiropractic, nutritional, and kinesiological disciplines of medicine.[4] I was really impressed when I saw her bowel movements change just a couple of days after the treatment. This technique is helpful because the AP treats the condition instead of completely eliminating the allergen so that the child is able to incorporate the food into his or her diet.

Don't panic when your child has a fever. Fevers are very common in children, especially in the first years when their immune systems are still developing. The way the body kills a virus or bacteria naturally is by raising the temperature in the body so that the agent cannot survive in it anymore. "Fever represents a universal, ancient, and usually beneficial response to infection, and its suppression under most circumstances has few, if any, demonstrable benefits. On the other hand, some harmful effects have been shown to occur as a result of suppressing fever…widespread use of antipyretics should not be encouraged either in developing countries or in industrial societies."[5] We go against our body in its war against the virus whenever we try to lower a fever. Research teaches us that allowing a fever to run its course "will actually strengthen the immune system in the long run"[6] and that "the powerful effects of a fever will even elevate your bodies' defense from cancer."[7]

Natural Remedies and Supplements for Fevers

None of us want our kids to have a fever or get sick, so here's what you can do. Make sure your child is properly hydrated by nursing or giving him or her plenty of water. Consider getting these natural supplements and remedies before rushing to the pharmacy to buy an over-the-counter drug:

- Carlson's Cod Liver Oil ($23): two doses per day.
- InForce Immune Builder ($32): Open a capsule and put a small amount under the tongue.
- Vitamin C+ Bio Fizz by Designs for Health ($29): One teaspoon has 2,569 grams of Vitamin C and it contains Xylitol, instead of sugar or artificial sweeteners.
- Children's ACF Immune Support ($17)
- Calcium Lactate by Standard Process ($10): Dissolve 2 capsules in water.
- Homemade vegetable juices: Try a carrot, beet, celery, and spinach juice. The carrot and beet will make it sweet. Add radishes to treat mucous, and garlic or ¼ small onion to add immune boosting properties.
- My friend Carey's foot balm garlic socks. You need two tablespoons of coconut oil, seven drops of tea tree oil, seven drops of lavender oil, seven drops of thieves oil, and about three garlic cloves minced into a paste. Mix all ingredients together and rub on the feet then cover with two pairs of socks. You may have to wait until your child is asleep to do this!

I keep the InForce, Vitamin C, and fish oil in stock. They are all available on Amazon. I also use them for my husband, older kids, and myself in a higher dosage. It is important to go as natural as possible when fighting a disease in light of the growing studies showing the dangers of Tylenol and Motrin in both pregnant women[8] and children.[9] Different studies show that the more a fever is suppressed by anti-fever drugs, the more difficult it is for the person to overcome the illness.[10] Lastly, avoid sugars because high amounts of it suppress the immune system. You want to make it as easy as possible for your child's body to heal.

It may be hard to manage the pressure from loved ones telling you to give Tylenol and Motrin, etc. Focus within (just like when birthing) and tune out opposing views. It's helpful to have a support system that will pray and encourage you along the way.

How to Avoid a Febrile Seizure

Febrile seizures are convulsion in young children caused by fevers.[11] There is a misconception that all seizures are the same and that all seizures may cause brain damage. The body will usually not reach a damaging temperature during naturally occurring fevers.[12] Doctors often tell parents that these events are benign and don't cause brain damage with the exception of prolonged febrile status epilepticus, which is rare.[13]

MedLine Plus, an online resource produced by the United States National Library of Medicine, states that, "Although a fever signals that a battle might be going on in the body, the fever is fighting for, not against, the person. Brain damage from a fever generally will not occur unless the fever is over 107.6°F (42°C). Untreated fevers caused by infection will seldom go over 105°F unless the child is overdressed or trapped in a hot place."[14]

Even though I know fevers are natural, I don't want Bella or any of my children to ever have a high fever or another seizure. Here is some information to help you navigate the fever naturally:

Watch out for changes in temperatures. Febrile seizures happen from sudden spikes in temperatures and not necessarily from high fevers or high body temperature.[15] Our kitchen area—where Bella was when she got the seizure—gets very hot in the afternoon. Be aware of the room or car temperature, especially during hot days, and keep a thermometer on hand to check for temperature changes.

Keep your child hydrated. Water is fundamental for keeping your body healthy and your immune system working. Your body can manage to be without food for 30-40 days, but can only go without water for two to three days.[16] I wish I told Ana to keep Bella hydrated and watch out for a fever. Ana told me that Bella asked for water repeatedly right before she had the seizure. She knew she needed it. Make sure to keep your

children hydrated whenever they are fighting a disease. Do not give them Gatorade or other sports drinks that contain sugars or artificial ingredients. Coconut water is a healthy alternative to water and actually hydrates more than water because of its high concentration of electrolytes.

Try color puncture. Color puncture is an alternative medicine practice where colored lights are directed in high intensity to acupuncture points in the body in order to promote healing and better health.[17] My friend, Samantha L., came to my house daily to perform color puncture on Bella while she healed from the febrile seizure. We always took her temperature before and after the color puncture, and her temperature always improved immediately after the treatment. You can learn more at *colorpuncture.org*.

Vitamin C showers and baths. We have a Vitamin C shower filter at home and tablets that neutralize the chlorine in water. You can find both of them on Amazon. Eliminating chloride from your water may even increase your immunity, since you are not continually being exposed to chloride through your skin. When Bella's fever got too high, I bathed her in lukewarm water that was colder than her body temperature, but not so cold that it would shock her body.

Supplement with calcium lactate. The fever or febrile seizure occurs when the body warms the muscles around bones in order to draw out ionized calcium and activate the white blood cells so that they can defend the body against the virus or infection. Ionized calcium is the active calcium in the blood. Unlike the serum calcium, which is attached to proteins, ionized calcium floats freely in the blood moving in and out of cells to enable actions or reactions.[18] "Calcium lactate is regarded as a good source of ionizable calcium to utilize in overcoming and/or preventing calcium deficits and thus fever and febrile seizures."[19] There no longer is a need for the fever because the body recognizes the abundance of the free calcium. Calcium lactate pills or raw milk are a good source because pasteurization in conventional milk destroys the calcium lactate. Dr. Lisa recommends treating fevers with two tablets of calcium lactate pills made by Standard Process. You can dissolve them in distilled water. Chlorine or fluoride will affect their efficacy. You can give your child the calcium lactate as a preventive measure when fever is present or as an emergency aid in case a seizure occurs.

How to React if a Seizure Occurs

If a seizure occurs, place your child on his or her side and let the seizure pass. This is what Ana did. She described Bella's seizure as a temper tantrum but with uncontrolled movements.

Most febrile seizures pass very fast, after a minute or two, while others can last for over fifteen minutes.[20] The paramedics that responded to our 911 call told us that Bella did not have to go to the hospital to treat the febrile seizure. Febrile seizures don't normally require additional examinations or blood evaluations.[21] Most children outgrow febrile seizures by age five, and few children have more than three febrile seizures in their lifetime. Research also shows that the number of febrile seizures is not related to a future risk of epilepsy.[22]

Baby Products I Love

Table 14.1 lists products I use frequently after researching and trying many others.

The majority of these products are available on Amazon for a 20% discount if you use the "Subscribe and Save" option. Amazon Mom can really save you money and trips to the store. I do not receive compensation for any subscriptions or for endorsing any of these products—I just think they are wonderful.

The Road Less Traveled

Remember my friend Ana's story—how she wished someone told her about other methods while she was stuck in a snowball of increasing medication dosages. Gabriel could hardly stay awake in school from the effects of the medication that controlled his seizures. But they didn't know there was another route.

TABLE 14.1 PRODUCTS I LOVE

Diapers	Seventh Generation Chlorine Free Diapers from Newborn and Beyond: overnight and pull-ups (approx. $40/month supply). I especially like their fit.
Wipes	Seventh Generation ($13/384 Count).
Diaper Rash and Moisturizer	I use organic extra virgin coconut oil from Carrington Farms and Nutiva (approx. $15). Coconut oil is great to moisturize and treat diaper rashes and mosquito bites. For a heavier cream, you can use NOW Foods Raw Shea Butter 7-ounce ($8).
Baby Soap/Shampoo	Earth Mama-Angel Baby Organic Angel Baby Shampoo & Body Wash in Natural Orange Vanilla ($10). I especially like that it is foam and smells great!
Conditioner/Detangler	Little Twig in Happy Tangerine 8.5 Ounces ($12.50).
Laundry Detergent	Seventh Generation Baby Natural 4X Laundry Detergent 32 fl oz ($13), especially in the beginning when their skin is so sensitive.
Mesh Feeder	This is great when you are introducing foods to your baby. I use Munchkin Fresh Food Feeder ($4).

You are now at the beginning of a new journey—at a crossroad. The road you take has the potential to affect the rest of your family's course. How will you approach your baby's health? Will you take the more popular conventional route—where symptoms are treated through medications with harmful side effects? Or will you take the one less traveled—the original road that has led humanity to health for centuries through healing the body instead of numbing the senses?

I chose the one less traveled and, like Robert Frost said, "that has made all the difference."[23]

Action Step: Share this book with someone you love.

I will share this book with: _____

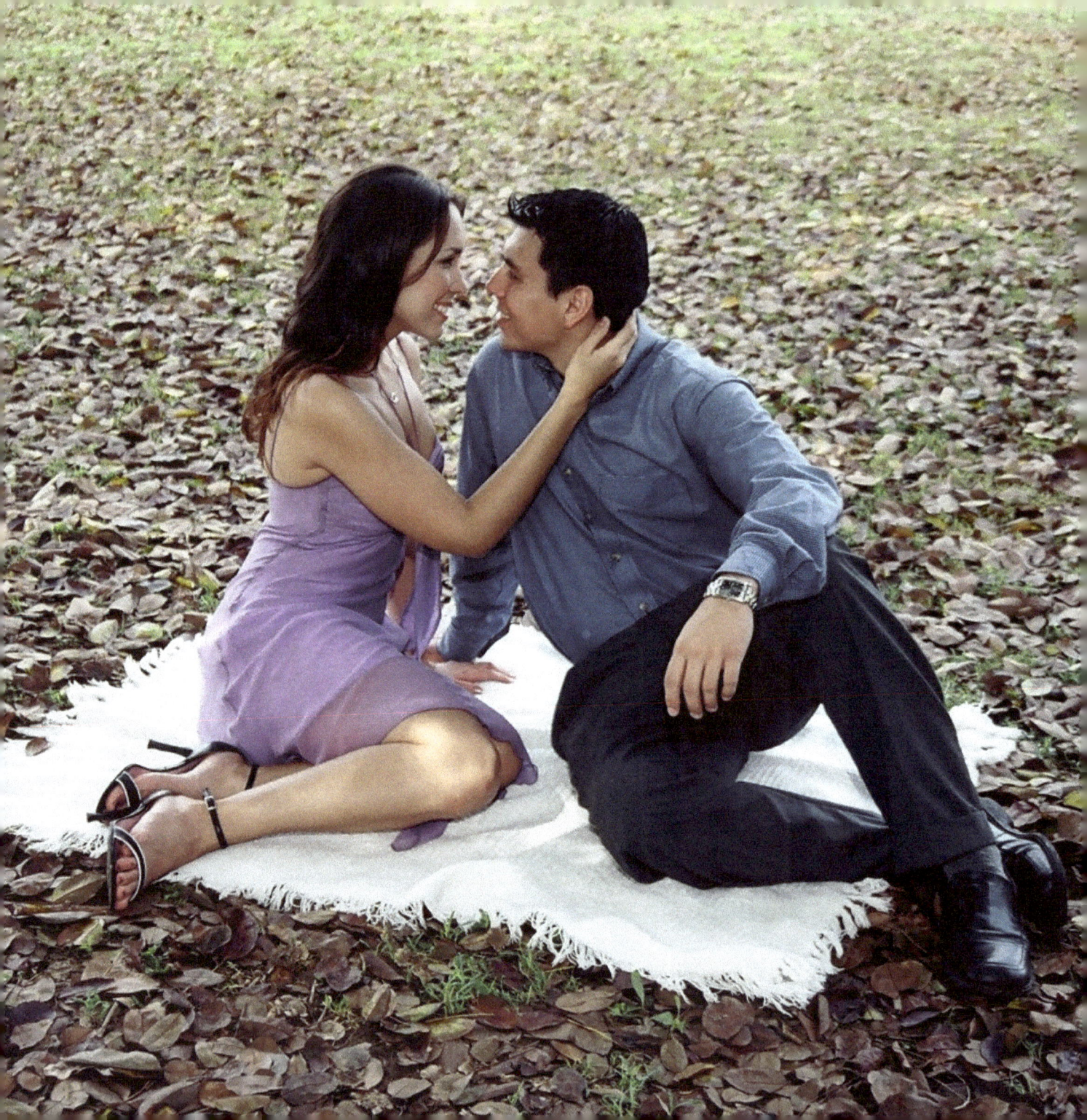

Epilogue: Perspective of a Skeptical Husband

by Joan Carlos Wizel

First, let me say a word to the women, from a husband's perspective.

When I think about this book and its message of a healthy pregnancy, I'm reminded of life with Christ. Stay with me. Living a Christian life does not mean you'll have a pain-free, struggle-free, or even illness-free life. It does mean that you will live your best possible pregnancy. You will be comforted in pain; you will have guidance in your struggles; and you will have hope in your illness. Much in the same way, following my wife's advice will not guarantee you a pain-free pregnancy full of rainbows and roses. In fact, I have seen some of the women discussed in this book go through their fair share of struggles in their pregnancies and post-pregnancy experiences (my wife included). But heeding to her advice will help you have your best possible pregnancy. The knowledge you'll gain from this book will give you the comfort, guidance, and confidence to sculpt your path through the very intricate process that is pregnancy.

Now, if you bought this book and are making your husband read this epilogue, spare him the first couple of paragraphs and start him off here—a word for the guys:

Don't picture me wrongly. I am not a free spirit. I am not a vegetarian. I am not a die-hard gym goer or calories-watcher kind of guy. And I was quite careless for a long time before my wife started her detox from the unhealthy. I had the eating habits of Homer Simpson. However, I did my fair share of exercise in the form of sports and was never obese, even though I did put on more extra weight than a healthy pregnant woman may put on during pregnancy after I started working full-time and stopped playing soccer. Fortunately, I have since dropped most of it.

I am a typical family man. I like sports (soccer is my fix), food (Churrasco? I'm in!), snacks (Cheetos are my favorite), and long, sleepy mornings on the weekends. You know—the good things in life. But I've had a first row ticket to this admirable transformation my wife has gone through, and I've been on the edge of my seat throughout the show. I've also been inevitably affected by it and have become a part of it along the way.

Sure, I thought it all sounded like hyperbolized, you're-gonna-die propaganda at first. You probably did too. I've discovered it isn't. You may not care much about it working or not right now.

But we all know that our wives conspire among themselves and there's no stopping them once they jump on a particular bandwagon. So our choice is limited: fall in line hoping it will be manageable (I know this is our hope for most of the craziness our wives put us through) or live bitterly in rebellion. And after having lived out the stuff in this book, my message is that it's not only manageable, but also actually enjoyable. You'll feel better for it too. Just give it a chance.

Lastly, a word of caution: don't forget about our role as moderators in this as in any other journey our lovely wives take us on. She may want to go all-in, all at once, which may not gel well with our man-wiring. The process has some built-in speed bumps already, but you may want to apply some light breaks throughout the curves on the road to make it a smooth ride for all. If you're doubtful about any aspect, have your wife explain it to you. It will build up her knowledge and confidence and will give you the comfort of knowing that it's important to her, so it should be important to you. And it's okay to be open but still have some limitations. For example, I drew the line at coffee enemas (see Chapter 1), no matter what the benefits may be.

In the end, I hope you feel the same way I do: immensely proud of your wife, comforted by the conviction that you are contributing to the overall well-being of your babies and family, and happy with your healthier life.

About the Author

Maria Andrea Wizel is a successful professional and entrepreneur turned health blogger and is dedicated to educating people about true health. Maria enjoys coaching women in all stages of pregnancy, including those preparing to conceive. Maria has been married to her high school sweetheart, JC, for ten years and they live in Miami, Florida. They became parents in 2009 when they adopted their two older kids. Since then, she has had two healthy pregnancies and natural childbirths.

Maria serves as the Director of Human Resources at her church, Calvary Fellowship, and provides consulting services to companies seeking to improve their human resources and marketing practices.

Maria has a Bachelor's degree in Business from the University of Puerto Rico, where she graduated with honors, and a Master's degree in Business Administration from the University of Miami, where she earned an Academic Excellence Award. She also completed an Executive Leadership program at Harvard University.

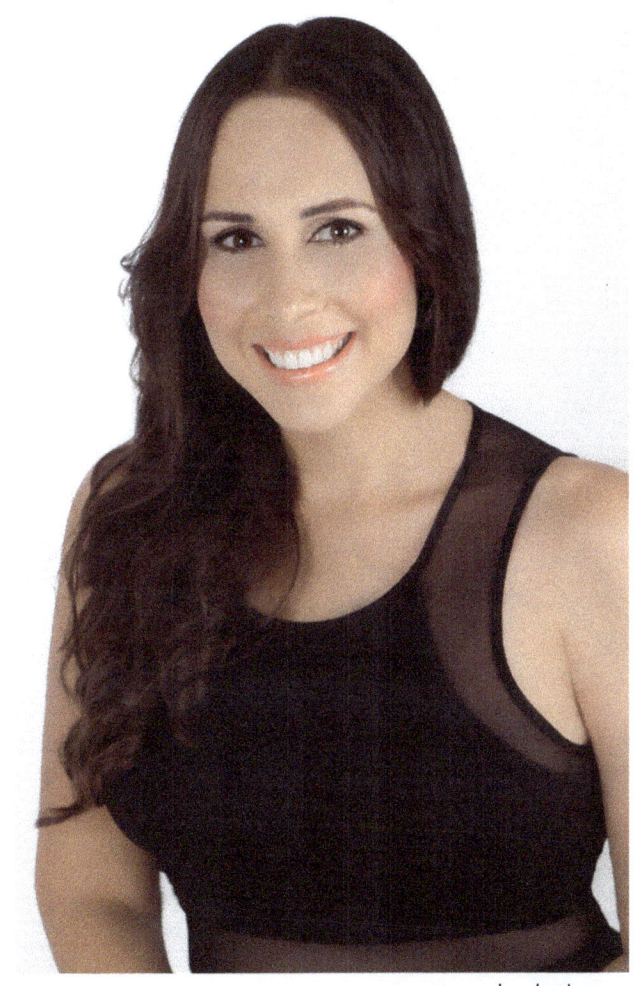

www.mariawizel.com

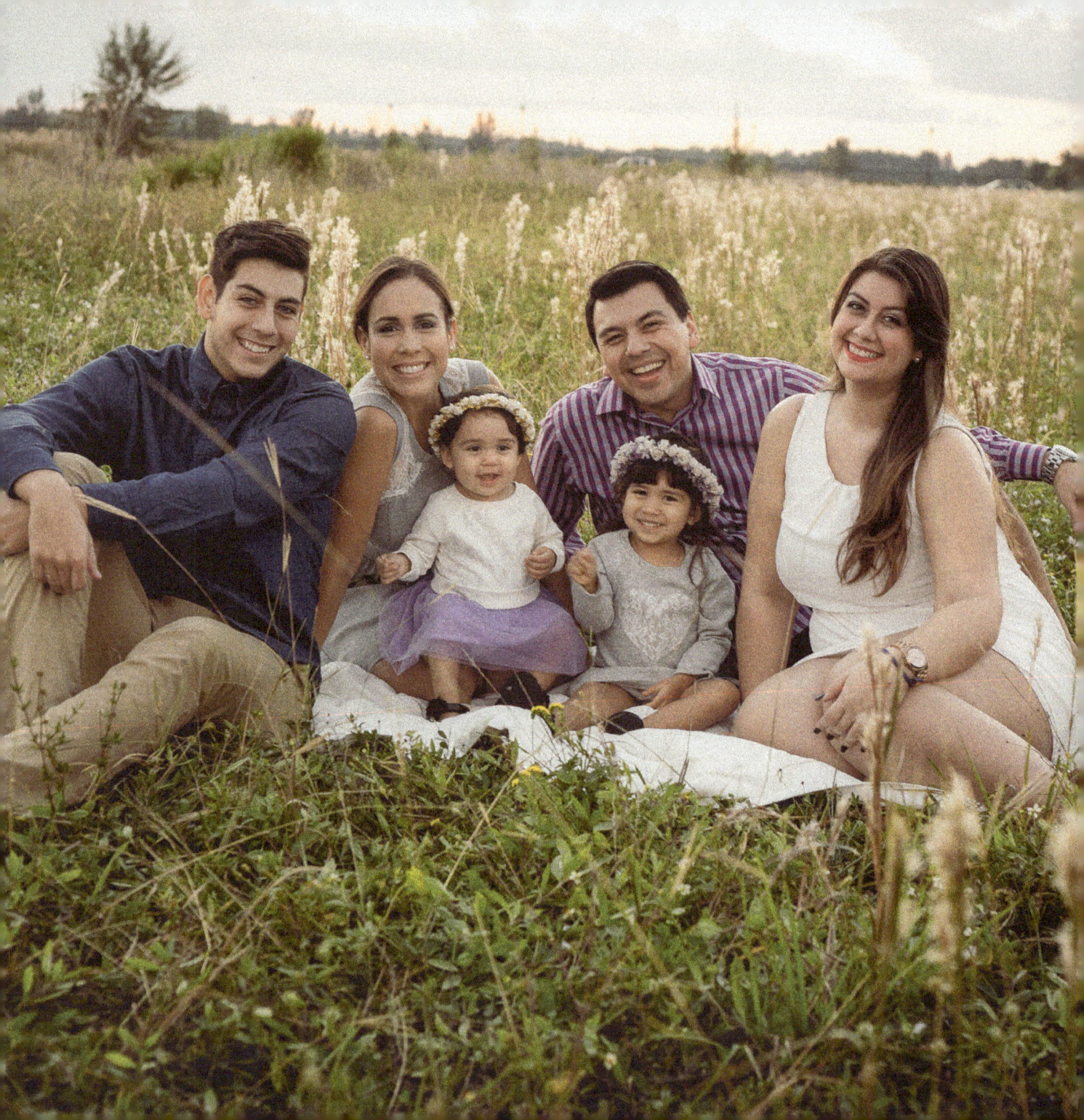

Endnotes

CHAPTER 1

1. Michael W. Smith, vocal performance of "Breath," by Marie Barnett, *Worship*, Reunion Records, CL 10025, compact disc, 2001.

2. Condoms, rhythm, and/or withdrawal (also known as "pull-out") are good back-up methods during your detox.

3. *Fat, Sick, and Nearly Dead*, directed by Joe Cross and Kurt Engfehr (2010; Reboot Media, 2011), DVD.

4. Suzy Cohen, "Coffee Enemas Are Not A Pain In The Butt," Dear Pharmacist. *Ocla Star Banner*, July 9, 2013, http://www.ocala.com/article/20130709/COLUMNISTS/130709758?Title=Coffee-enemas-are-not-a-pain-in-the-butt.

5. Rebecca Smith, "Obese Pregnant Women Have More Complicated Births: Research," *The Telegraph*, January 26, 2011, http://www.telegraph.co.uk/health/healthnews/8280720/Obese-pregnant-women-have-more-complicated-births-research.html.

6. Cynthia Aranow, MD, "Vitamin D and The Immune System," *Journal of Investigative Medicine* 59, no. 6 (August 2011): 881-886, doi: 10.231/JIM.0b013e31821b8755.

7. "12 Ways To Get Your Daily Vitamin D," Ella Quittner, Health Magazine, accessed February 7, 2014, http://www.health.com/health/gallery/0,,20504538,00.html.

8. "Magnesium In Your Pregnancy Diet," Baby Center, accessed February 7, 2014, http://www.babycenter.com/0_magnesium-in-your-pregnancy-diet_659.bc.

9. Ibid.

10. Robert Frost, "The Road Not Taken," lines 18-20.

11. "Does Microwaving Food Remove Its Nutritional Value?," Bob Barnett, CNN.com, last modified February 1, 2014, http://www.cnn.com/2014/01/21/health/upwave-microwaving-food/.

12. "Microwave Ovens and Health," FDA.gov, last modified October 8, 2014, http://www.fda.gov/radiation-emittingproducts/resourcesforyouradiationemittingproducts/ucm252762.htm.

13. "Why Therapeutic Benefits of Coffee Do Not Apply to Pregnant Women," Dr. Joseph Mercola, Mercola.com, accessed February 7, 2014, http://articles.mercola.com/sites/articles/archive/2014/02/03/coffee-in-pregnancy.aspx.

14. "Light Drinking During Pregnancy," NOFAS.org, accessed February 7, 2014, http://www.nofas.org/light-drinking/.

15. Ibid.

16. "Harmful Effects of Excess Sugar," AskDrSears.com, accessed February 7, 2014, http://www.askdrsears.com/topics/feeding-eating/family-nutrition/sugar/harmful-effects-excess-sugar.

17. Ibid.

18. "Study: Taking Just a Little Too Much Tylenol Each Time Can Be Deadly," Maia Szalavitz, Time.com, last modified November 23, 2011, http://healthland.time.com/2011/11/23/study-taking-too-much-tylenol-each-time-can-be-deadly/.

19. "Cough Suppressant Linked to Birth Defects," Mercola.com, last modified January 02, 2008, http://articles.mercola.com/sites/articles/archives/2008/01/02/cough-suppressants.aspx.

20. "The Health Consequences of Secondhand Smoke (Involuntary Exposure to Tobacco Smoke)," University of Miami, accessed February 7, 2014, http://www6.miami.edu/communications/smokefree/secondhand-smoke-effects.pdf.

21. "Pregnant Women: Secondhand Smoke Can Harm Your Unborn Baby," Leslie Wade, *The Chart* (blog), *CNN.com*, last modified March 7, 2011, http://thechart.blogs.cnn.com/2011/03/07/pregnant-women-secondhand-smoke-can-harm-your-unborn-baby/.

22. "What Is Spina Bifida?," Spina Bifida Association, accessed February 7, 2014, http://www.spinabifidaassociation.org/site/c.evKRI7OXIoJ8H/b.8277225/k.5A79/What_is_Spina_Bifida.htm.

23. "Is Fluoride In Our Water a Mistake?," Philip Frazer, Pure Water Products, LLC, accessed February 7, 2014, http://www.purewaterproducts.com/articles/fluoride-mistake.

24. "MSG: Is This Silent Killer Lurking in Your Kitchen Cabinets," Dr. Joseph Mercola, Mercola.com, last modified April 21, 2009, http://articles.mercola.com/sites/articles/archive/2009/04/21/msg-is-this-silent-killer-lurking-in-your-kitchen-cabinets.aspx.

25. Theresa Bonner, "Know Your MSG," Enlightened Nourishment (blog), January 6, 2014, http://enlightenednourishment.com/2014/01/06/know-your-msg/.

26. "Types of Products That Contain MSG," TruthInLabeling.org, accessed February 7, 2014, http://www.truthinlabeling.org/II.WhereISMSG.html.

27. Anne Mullens, "Parabens: What Are They, and Are They Really That Bad?," Best Health Magazine, Summer 2008, http://www.besthealthmag.ca/look-great/beauty/parabens-what-are-they-and-are-they-really-that-bad.

28. Ibid.

29. "Tips to Avoid Toxic Chemicals Before, During, and After Pregnancy," Women's Voices For The Earth, accessed February 7, 2014, http://womensvoices.org/avoid-toxic-chemicals/pregnancy/.

30. Ibid.

31. "Pregnancy, Foods and Supplements: The Good, The Bad and The Ugly," Webster Kehr, CancerTutor.com, last modified February 19, 2014, http://www.cancertutor.com/pregnant/.

32. "Tips to Avoid Toxic Chemicals Before, During, and After Pregnancy," Women's Voices For The Earth, accessed February 7, 2014, http://womensvoices.org/avoid-toxic-chemicals/pregnancy/.

33. Flu Vaccine Exposed," Mercola.com, last modified September 26, 2009, http://articles.mercola.com/sites/articles/archive/2009/09/26/flu-vaccine-exposed.aspx.

Chapter 3

1. "Obese Pregnant Women Have More Complicated Births: Research," Rebecca Smith, *The Telegraph*, last modified January 26, 2011, http://www.telegraph.co.uk/health/healthnews/8280720/Obese-pregnant-women-have-more-complicated-births.html.

2. Dr. Miriam Stoppard, *Bonding Before Birth* (New York: DK Publishing, 2008), 11-12.

3. Anna Sapone, Karen M. Lammers, Vinncenzo Casolaro, Marcella Cammarota, Maria Teresa Giuliano, Mario De Rosa, Rosita Stefanile, Giuseppe Mazzarella, Carlo Tolone, Maria Itria Russo, Pasquale Esposito, Franca Ferraraccio, Maria Carteni, Gabriele Riegler, Laura de Magistris, and Alessio Fasano, "Divergence of Gut Permeability and Mucosal Immune Gene Expression In Two Gluten-Associated Conditions: Celiac Disease and Gluten Sensitivity," *BMC Medicine* 9, no. 23 (2011), doi: 10.1186/1741-7015-9-23.

4. G. Vighi, F. Marcucci, L. Sensi, G. Di Cara, and F. Frati, "Allergy and The Gastrointestinal System," *Clinical & Experimental Immunology* 153, no. S1 (July 21, 2008): 3-6, doi: 10.1111/j.1365-2249.2008.03713.x.

5. "Gluten: The Whole Story," Frank Lipman, DrFrankLipman.com, accessed February 14, 2014, http://www.drfranklipman.com/gluten-the-whole-story/.

6. "What Does the Small Intestine Do?," Dr. Ananya Mandal, MD, News Medical, last modified November 1, 2013, http://www.news-medical.net/health/What-Does-the-Small-Intestine-Do.aspx.

7. "Coeliac Disease and Gluten Sensitivity," Better Health Channel, last modified May 2014, http://www.betterhealth.vic.gov.au/bhcv2/bhcarticles.nsf/pages/Coeliac_disease_and_gluten_sensitivity?open.

8. Jonas F. Ludvigsson, MD, PhD, Abraham Reichenberg, PhD, Christina M. Hultman, PhD, and Joseph A. Murray, MD, "A Nationwide Study of the Association Between Celiac Disease and the Risk of Autistic Spectrum Disorders," *JAMA Psychiatry* 70, no. 11 (November 2013): 1224-1230, doi: 10.1001/jamapsychiatry.2013.2048.

9. "Shoppers Guide to Pesticides in Produce," University of North Carolina Wilmington, accessed February 14, 2014, http://uncw.edu/healthservices/documents/EWG_pesticide.pdf.

10. "Pesticides in the News," Organic Consumers Association, last modified July 22, 1999, http://www.organicconsumers.org/old_articles/Toxic/rach660.php.

11. Thierry Vrain, "Former Pro-GMO Scientist Speaks Out On The Real Dangers of Genetically Engineered Food, *The Food Revolution Network* (blog), May 11, 2013, http://foodrevolution.org/blog/former-pro-gmo-scientist/.

12. Gilles-Eric Séralini, Emilie Clair, Robin Mesnage, Steeve Gress, Nicloas Defarge, Manuela Malatesta, Didier Hennequin, and Joël Spiroux de Vendômois, "Long Term Toxicity of A Roundup Herbicide and A Roundup-Tolerant Genetically Modified Maize," *Food and Chemical Toxicology* 50, no. 11 (November 2012): 4221-4231.

    Joël Spiroux de Vendômois, François Roullier, Dominique Cellier, and Gilles-Eric Séralini, "A Comparison of The Effects of Three GM Corn Varieties on Mammalian Health," *International Journal of Biological Sciences* 5, no. 7 (2009): 706-726, doi: 10.7150/ijbs.5.706.

13. "6 Easy Ways To Avoid GMO's," Food Matters, last modified August 13, 2013, http://foodmatters.tv/articles-1/6-easy-ways-to-avoid-gmos.

14. "Monsanto is a multinational agricultural biotechnology corporation based in the United States. They are the world's leading producer of Roundup®, a herbicide with the active ingredient glyphosate."

    "Who is Monsanto," WhoIsMonsanto.com, accessed February 14, 2014, http://whoismonsanto.com. Throughout its history, Monsanto has developed chemical products which have eventually become controversial or been banned.

15. Esther E. McGinnis, Mary H. Meyer, and Alan G. Smith, letter to the editor, *The Plant Cell* 22, no. 6 (June 2010): 1653-1657, doi: 10.1105/tpc.110.077198.

16. "The Top 20 GMO Foods and Ingredients to Avoid," Global Healing Center (Blog), last modified July 24, 2013, http://www.globalhealingcenter.com/natural-health/top-20-gmo-foods-and-ingredients-to-avoid/.

17. "What Is Neurotoxicity?," William J. Rea, M.D. and Kaye Kilburn, M.D., The American Environmental Health Foundation, accessed February 14, 2014, http://www.aehf.com/articles/Defin-neurotox.html.

18. "A Sweet Problem: Princeton Researchers Find That High-fructose Corn Syrup Prompts Considerably More Weight Gain," Hilary Parker, Princeton University, last modified March 22, 2010, http://www.princeton.edu/main/news/archive/S26/91/22K07/.

    "Research Indicates Risks of Consuming High Fructose Corn Syrup," University of Oxford, last modified November 28, 2012, http://www.ox.ac.uk/news/2012-11-28-research-indicates-risks-consuming-high-fructose-corn-syrup.

19. Javier A. Magaña-Gómez, Guillermo López Cervantes, Gloria Yepiz-Plascencia, and

Ana M. Calderón De La Barca, "Pancreatic Response of Rats Fed Genetically Modified Soybean," *Journal of Applied Toxicology* 28, no. 2 (2008): 217-26, doi:10.1002/jat.1319.

20. "6 Easy Ways To Avoid GMO's," Food Matters, last modified August 13, 2013, http://www.foodmatters.tv/articles-1/6-easy-ways-to-avoid-gmos.

21. Hugh J. Beckie, K. Neil Harker, Anne Légère, Malcom J. Morrison, Ginette Séguin-Swartz, and Kevin C. Falk, "GM Canola: The Canadian Experience," *Farm Policy Journal* 8, no. 1 (Autumn 2011): 43-49.

22. Eugenia Venneria, Simone Fanasca, Giovanni Monastra, Enrico Finotti, Roberto Ambra, Elena Azzini, Alessandra Durazzo, Maria Stella Foddai, and Giuseppe Maiani, "Assessment of the Nutritional Values of Genetically Modified Wheat, Corn, and Tomato Crops," *Journal of Agricultural and Food Chemistry* 56, no. 19 (October 08, 2008): 9206-214, doi:10.1021/jf8010992.

23. "FP967 ('Triffid') Flax Has Been Grown Illegally in Canada and Exported Around the Globe," GM Contamination Register, accessed February 14, 2014, http://www.gmcontaminationregister.org/index.php?content=nw_detail1.

24. "The Top 20 GMO Foods and Ingredients to Avoid," Global Healing Center, last modified July 24, 2013, http://www.global-healingcenter.com/natural-health/top-20-gmo-foods-and-ingredients-to-avoid/.

25. "GM Food Toxins Found In the Blood of 93% of Unborn BabiesSean," Poulter, Health, DailyMail.co.uk, last modified May 20, 2011, http://www.dailymail.co.uk/health/article-1388888/GM-food-toxins-blood-93-unborn-babies.html.

26. Ibid.

27. Aifric O'Sullivan, Xuan He, Elizabeth M. S. Mcniven, Neill W. Haggarty, Bo Lönnerdal, and Carolyn M. Slupsky, "Early Diet Impacts Infant Rhesus Gut Microbiome, Immunity, and Metabolism," *Journal of Proteome Research* 12, no. 6 (2013): 2833-845, doi:10.1021/pr4001702.

28. "Foods With Most and Least Pesticides," Food Democracy, last modified November 8, 2007, https://fooddemocracy.wordpress.com/2007/11/08/460/.

29. "PLU Codes," Snopes.com, last modified May 30, 2013, http://www.snopes.com/food/prepare/produce.asp#k5E3CfMqzRSoSC8x.99.

30. "Six Easy Steps To Avoid Common Genetically Modified Foods," Jonathan Benson, Natural News, last modified August 10, 2013, http://www.naturalnews.com/041573_GMOs_avoid_foods.html##ixzz2tQbnL3Cd.

31. "PLU Codes," Snopes.com, last modified May 30, 2013, http://www.snopes.com/food/prepare/produce.asp#k5E3CfMqzRSoSC8x.99.

32. http://www.TowerGarden.com/.

Chapter 4

1. "How To Treat Gestational Diabetes," American Diabetes Association, last modified April 29, 2014, http://www.diabetes.org/diabetes-basics/gestational/how-to- treat-gestational.html. The American Diabetes Association recommends exercise as a helpful therapy for women who are at risk.

2. "Exercise: 7 Benefits of Regular Physical Activity," The Mayo Clinic, last modified February 5, 2014, http://www.mayoclinic.org/healthy-living/fit-ness/in-depth/exercise/art-20048389 exercise/art-20046495.

3. Guistino Varrassi, Carmello Bazzano, and W. Thomas Edwards, "Effects Of Physical Activity On Maternal Plasma Beta-Endorphin Levels and Perception of Labor Pain," *American Journal of Obstetrics and Gynecology* 160, no. 3 (1989): 707-12, doi:10.1016/S0002-9378(89)80065-1.

4. "Exercise and Depression," WebMD, last modified February 19, 2014, http://www.webmd.com/depression/guide/exercise-depression.

5. Sarah McGraw Crow 10 Secrets to an Easier Labor Parents.com http://www.parents.com/pregnancy/giving-birth/labor-and-delivery/10-secrets-to-an-easier-labor/.

6. Guistino Varrassi, Carmello Bazzano, and W. Thomas Edwards, "Effects Of Physical Activity On Maternal Plasma Beta-Endorphin Levels and Perception of Labor Pain," *American Journal of Obstetrics and Gynecology* 160, no. 3 (1989): 707-12, doi:10.1016/S0002-9378(89)80065-1.

7. "10 Secrets To An Easier Labor," Sarah McGraw Crow, Parents.com, accessed March 16, 2014, http://www.parents.com/pregnancy/giving-birth/labor-and-delivery/10-secrets-to-an-easier-labor/.

8. C.R. Beckmann and C.A. Beckmann, "Effect of a Structured Antepartum Exercise Program on Pregnancy and Labor Outcome in Primiparas," *The Journal of Reproductive Medicine* 35, no.7 (1990): 704-709.

9. James F. Clapp III, M.D., "The Course of Labor after Endurance Exercise during Pregnancy," *American Journal of Obstetrics and Gynecology* 163, no. 6 (1990): 1799-805, doi:10.1016/0002-9378(90)90753-T.

10. Ibid.

    277 total pregnancy days (39 ½ weeks) ± 6 days for the women that exercised versus 282 (40 weeks and a couple of days) total pregnancy days ± 6 days for the women that stopped.

11. Colette Bouchez, "Exercise During Pregnancy: Myth vs. Fact," WebMD, last modified February 6, 2009, http://www.webmd.com/baby/features/exercise-during-pregnancy-myth-vs-fact?page=2.

Chapter 5

1. Charles M. Schulz and Gordon Volke, *Charlie Brown's Little Book of Wisdom*, Partridge Green: Ravette, 2001.

2. "Poor sleep quality and quantity during pregnancy can disrupt normal immune processes and lead to lower birth weights and other complications, finds a University of Pittsburgh School of Medicine study…" "Poor Sleep In Pregnancy Can Disrupt The Immune System and Cause Birth-Related Complications," ScienceDaily, July 17, 2013, http://www.sciencedaily.com/releases/2013/07/130717164725.htm.

3. "The Virtues of Napping," Reader'sDigest.ca, accessed June 28, 2014, http://www.readersdigest.ca/health/healthy-living/virtues-napping/.

4. "Power Naps: Napping Benefits, Length, and Tips," Jennifer Soong, WebMD, accessed June 28, 2014, http://www.m.webmd.com/a-to-z-guides/features/the-secret-and-surprising-power-of-naps.

5. Shao-Yu Tsai, Jou-Wei Lin, Lu-Ting Kuo, Chien-Nan Lee, and Carol A. Landis, "Nighttime Sleep, Daytime Napping, and Labor Outcomes in Healthy Pregnant Women in Taiwan," *Research in Nursing & Health* 36, no. 6 (2013): 612-22, doi:10.1002/nur.21568.

    A study examined the associations of nighttime and daytime sleep during the third trimester of pregnancy with labor duration and risk of cesarean deliveries in a convenience sample of 120 nulliparous women who completed sleep-related questionnaires and wore wrist actigraphs for up to 7 days. Nap duration and 24-hour sleep duration were inversely associated with labor duration in women with vaginal delivery.

6. "The Virtues of Napping," Reader'sDigest.ca, June 28, 2014, http://www.readers-

digest.ca/health/healthy-living/virtues-napping/.

7. "Napping May Not Be Such a No-No," Harvard Medical School, accessed June 28, 2014, http://www.health.harvard.edu/newsletters/Harvard_Health_Letter/2009/November/napping-may-not-be-such-a-no-no.

Chapter 6

1. "Naturopathic Medicine," Naturopathic Medicine for Cancer Treatment, accessed March 31, 2014, http://www.cancercenter.com/treatments/naturopathic-medicine/?source=GGLPS01&channel=paid%20search&c=paid%20search:Google:Top%20Terms:Exact:naturopathic+medicine:Exact&OVMTC=Exact&site=&creative=35207429601&OVKEY=naturopathic%20medicine&url_id=190111119&adpos=1s1&device=c&gclid=CJ2l28zxn-sICFQcxaQodL1UAFg.

2. "About Page," DrPaulGannon.com, accessed March 31, 2014, http://drpaulgannon.com/about-2#.UyxRYChBBH0.

3. "Iris Diagnosis," Health-Science-Spirit.com, accessed March 31, 2014, http://www.health-science-spirit.com/iris.diagnosis.html.

4. "BioMeridian Testing," BioMeridian Testing, accessed March 31, 2014, http://www.biomeridiantesting.com/.

Chapter 7

1. "External Cephalic Version (Version) for Breech Position," WebMD, last modified July 24, 2013, http://www.m.webmd.com/baby/external-cephalic-version-version-for-breech-position#tn8179.

Chapter 8

1. "How Workplace Chemicals Enter the Body," Canadian Centre for Occupational Health and Safety, last modified April 1, 2009, http://www.ccohs.ca/oshanswers/chemicals/how_chem.html.

2. http://www.ewg.org/skindeep/.

3. http://www.GoodGuide.com/.

4. "Bath Care and Shower Products," Mercola.com, accessed April 2, 2014, http://bath-care.mercola.com/.

5. "What Are the Harmful Ingredients in Toothpaste?," William Lynch, LIVESTRONG.COM, last modified March 12, 2014, http://www.livestrong.com/article/167101-what-are-the-harmful-ingredients-in-toothpaste/.

6. "Can Perineal Massage Help Me Avoid An Episiotomy?," BabyCenter.com, last modified December 2011, http://www.babycenter.com/404_can-perineal-massage-help-me-avoid-an-episiotomy_1955.bc.

7. "Do Your Kegels: A Kegel Exercise Primer," Whattoexpect.com, last modified October 23, 2013, http://www.whattoexpect.com/pregnancy/pregnancy-health/kegels.aspx.

8. "Stages of Pregnancy," Pregnancy, Women'sHealth.gov, last modified September 27, 2010, http://www.womenshealth.gov/pregnancy/you-are-pregnant/stages-of-pregnancy.html.

9. "Avoid Fetal 'Keepsake' Images, Heartbeat Monitors," FDA.gov, last modified, March 24, 2008, http://www.fda.gov/ForConsumers/ConsumerUpdates/ucm095508.htm.

10. Joachim W. Ellwart, Hans Brettel, and Lorenz O. Kober, "Cell Membrane Damage by Ultrasound at Different Cell Concentrations," *Ultrasound in Medicine & Biology* 14, no. 1 (1988): 43-50, doi:10.1016/0301-5629(88)90162-7.

11. "First Trimester," BabyCenter.com, accessed April 2, 2014, http://www.babycenter.com/pregnancy-growing-baby-weeks-2-13.

12. "Inside Your Womb," BabyCenter.com, accessed April 2, 2014, http://www.babycenter.com/fetal-development-inside-your-womb.

13. Ibid.

14. "Sex During Pregnancy: An Overview," BabyCenter.com, accessed April 2, 2014, http://www.babycenter.com/sex-during-pregnancy-overview.

15. "Your Three Trimester Guide To Pregnant Sex," Robin Elise Weiss, About.com, last modified November 27, 2014, http://pregnancy.about.com/od/sexuality/a/Pregnant-Sex.htm.

16. Ibid.

17. "Sex After The Birth," BabyCentre.co.uk, last modified May 2013, http://www.babycentre.co.uk/a536362/sex-after-the-birth.

Chapter 9

1. Christopher Bergland, "Cortisol: Why 'The Stress Hormone' Is Public Enemy No. 1," *The Athlete's Way* (blog), *Psychology Today*, January 22, 2013, http://www.psychologytoday.com/blog/the-athletes-way/201301/cortisol-why-the-stress-hormone-is-public-enemy-no-1.

2. Ibid.

3. "Stress and Anxiety," Health Guide, The New York Times, accessed June 21, 2014, http://www.nytimes.com/health/guides/symptoms/stress-and-anxiety/possible-complications.html.

4. "Progesterone Treatment to Prevent Preterm Birth," March of Dimes, accessed June

21, 2014, http://www.marchofdimes.org/pregnancy/progesterone-treatment-to-prevent-preterm-birth.aspx#.

5. Bea R.H. Bergh, Van Den, Eduard J.H. Mulder, Maarten Mennes, and Vivette Glover, "Antenatal Maternal Anxiety and Stress and the Neurobehavioural Development of the Fetus and Child: Links and Possible Mechanisms. A Review," *Neuroscience & Biobehavioral Reviews* 29, no. 2 (2005): 237-58, doi:10.1016/j.neubiorev.2004.10.007.

6. "Excessive Amniotic Fluid (polyhydramnios)," BabyCenter, last modified October 2014, http://www.babycenter.com/0_excessive-amniotic-fluid-polyhydramnios_1200199.bc.

7. P. K. Bergman Sarkar, N. M. Fisk, T. G. O'Connor, and V. Glover, "Ontogeny of Foetal Exposure to Maternal Cortisol Using Midtrimester Amniotic Fluid as a Biomarker," *Clinical Endocrinology* 66, no. 5 (2007): 636-40, doi:10.1111/j.1365-2265.2007.02785.x.

8. "Why It's Never Too Late To Show Love: The Essential Vitamin For Children," Miriam Stoppard, The Mirror, last modified December 10, 2012, http://www.mirror.co.uk/lifestyle/health/dr-miriam-stoppard-advice-love-1482343.

9. Ibid.

10. Natalie Grizenko, MD, Marie-Eve Fortier, PhD, Christin Zadorozny, Geeta Thakur, Norburt Schmitz, PhD, Renaud Duval, MD, and Ridha Joober, MD, PhD, "Maternal Stress During Pregnancy, ADHD Symptomatology in Children and Genotype: Gene-Environment Interaction," *Journal of the Canadian Academy of Child and Adolescent Psychiatry* 21, no. 1 (February 2012): 9-15.

11. Natalie Grizenko, MD, Yasaman Rajabieh Shayan, Anna Polotskaia, Marina Ter-Stepanian, and Ridha Joober, MD, PhD, "Relation of Maternal Stress During Pregnancy to Symptom Severity and Response to Treatment in Children with ADHD," *Journal of Psychiatry & Neuroscience* 33, no.1 (January 2008): 10-16.

12. Dr. Miriam Stoppard, *Bonding Before Birth* (New York: DK Publishing, 2008), 11.

13. "The Secret (and Surprising) Power of Naps," Jennifer Soong, WebMD, last modified November 29, 2011, http://www.webmd.com/balance/features/the-secret-and-surprising-power-of-naps?page=2.

14. "Why Worrying Is A Waste of Time," Greg Laurie, WND.com, last modified January 15, 2011, http://mobile.wnd.com/2011/01/251025/#xxSL3UVMM1hmvBA3.99.

Chapter 10

1. "Benefits of Breastmilk," AskDrSears, accessed May 26, 2014, http://www.askdrsears.com/topics/feeding-eating/breastfeeding/why-breast-is-best/how-human-milk-protects-babies-illness.

   Colostrum is the milk mothers produce in the first few days after birth, is especially rich in IgA, just at the time when the newborn is first exposed to the outside world and needs protection from germs and foreign substances entering his body. Colostrum also contains higher amounts of white blood cells and infection-fighting substances than mature milk.

2. "Weight Gain," Anne Smith, Breastfeeding Basics, last modified December 2013, http://www.breastfeedingbasics.com/articles/weight-gain.

3. "Average Weight Gain for Breastfed Babies," KellyMom, last modified August 14, 2011, http://kellymom.com/bf/normal/weight-gain/.

4. "Tongue-tie," South Hampton Children's Hospital, accessed May 26, 2014, http://www.uhs.nhs.uk/OurServices/Childhealth/Tonguetie/Tonguetie.aspx.

5. "Tongue-tie (ankyloglossia)," Mayo Clinic, last modified May 16, 2012, http://www.mayoclinic.org/diseases-conditions/tongue-tie/basics/definition/con-20035410?reDate=01122014.

6. "Breastfeeding Glossary of Terms with Medical Definitions," EMedicineHealth, accessed May 26, 2014, http://www.emedicinehealth.com/breastfeeding/glossary_em.htm.

7. "Alternative Feeding Methods," Donna Murray, Health, About.com, last modified, September 23, 2014, http://breastfeeding.about.com/od/problemssolutions/a/Alternative-Feeding-Methods.htm.

8. "Cue Feeding: Breastfeeding On Demand," Breastfeeding-Problems.com, accessed May 26, 2014, http://www.breastfeeding-problems.com/cue-feeding.html.

9. "U.S. Moms Don't Breast-Feed Long Enough.," Robin Eisner, ABC News, last modified June 07, 2014, http://abcnews.go.com/Health/story?id=117395.

10. "ABM Affirms Breastfeeding Beyond Infancy as the Biological Norm," *Breastfeeding Medicine* (blog), *Academy of Breastfeeding Medicine*, last modified May 15, 2012, https://bfmed.wordpress.com/2012/05/15/abm-affirms-breastfeeding-beyond-infancy-as-the-biological-norm/.

11. "Breastfeeding and the Use of Human Milk," *Pediatrics* 129, no. 3 (2012): E827-841, doi:10.1542/peds.2011-3552.

12. "The World Health Organization's Infant Feeding Recommendation," Nutrition Topics, The World Health Organization, accessed May 26, 2014, http://www.who.int/nutrition/topics/infantfeeding_recommendation/en/.

13. Ibid.

14. "Breastfeeding, Family Physicians Supporting (Position Paper)," Policies, American Academy of Family Physicians, accessed May 26, 2014, http://www.aafp.org/about/policies/all/breastfeeding-support.html.

15. "Breastfeeding Past Infancy: Fact Sheet," Kelly Bonyata, KellyMom, last modified July 26, 2011, http://kellymom.com/ages/older-infant/ebf-benefits/.

16. Joan Younger Meek, ed. with Winnie Yu, *New Mother's Guide to Breastfeeding*, 2nd ed. (New York: Bantam Books, 2011), 11.

17. Megan A. Moreno, Fred Furtner, and Frederick P. Rivara, "Breastfeeding as Obesity Prevention," *Archives of Pediatrics and Adolescent Medicine* 165, no. 8 (2011): 772, doi:10.1001/archpediatrics.2011.140.

18. Jo L. Freudenheim, James R. Marshall, Saxon Graham, Rosemary Laughlin, John E. Vena, Elisa Bandera, Paola Muti, Mya Swanson, and Takuma Nemoto, "Exposure to Breastmilk in Infancy and the Risk of Breast Cancer," *Epidemiology* 5, no. 3 (1994): 324-31, doi:10.1097/00001648-199405000-00011.

19. "Breastfeeding Past Infancy: Fact Sheet," Kelly Bonyata, KellyMom, last modified July 26, 2011, http://kellymom.com/ages/older-infant/ebf-benefits/.

20. A. Lucas, R. Morley, T.J. Cole, G. Lister, and C. Leeson-Payne, "Breast Milk and Subsequent Intelligence Quotient in Children Born Preterm," *The Lancet* 339, no. 8788 (1992): 261-64, doi:10.1016/0140-6736(92)91329-7. This study found that babies fed their mother's milk had a significantly higher IQ (rise of 8.3 points) at seven to eight years of age than those who were formula fed, even after adjusting for the mom's educational, social, and economic status.

21. Paulita Duazo, Josephine Avila, and Christopher W. Kuzawa, "Breastfeeding and Later Psychosocial Development in the Philippines," *American Journal of Human Biology* 22, no. 6 (2010): 725-30, doi:10.1002/ajhb.21073.

C. Baumgartner, "Psychomotor and social development of breast-fed and bottle-fed babies during their first year of life," *Acta Paediatrica Hungarica* 25, no. 4 (1984): 409-417.

22. Joan Younger Meek, ed. with Winnie Yu, *New Mother's Guide to Breastfeeding*, 2nd ed. (New York: Bantam Books, 2011), 13.

23. "Breastfeeding Benefits for Mom and Baby," Health & Baby Center, WebMD, last modified December 30, 2013, http://www.webmd.com/parenting/baby/nursing-basics.

24. Jo L. Freudenheim, James R. Marshall, Saxon Graham, Rosemary Laughlin, John E. Vena, Elisa Bandera, Paola Muti, Mya Swanson, and Takuma Nemoto, "Exposure to Breastmilk in Infancy and the Risk of Breast Cancer," *Epidemiology* 5, no. 3 (1994): 324-31, doi:10.1097/00001648-199405000-00011.

25. "ABM Affirms Breastfeeding Beyond Infancy as the Biological Norm," *Breastfeeding Medicine* (blog), *Academy of Breastfeeding Medicine*, last modified May 15, 2012, https://bfmed.wordpress.com/2012/05/15/abm-affirms-breastfeeding-beyond-infancy-as-the-biological-norm/.

26. "Exclusive Breastfeeding," Nutrition, WorldHealthOrganization, accessed May 26, 2014, http://www.who.int/nutrition/topics/exclusive_breastfeeding/en/.

27. "Breastfeeding Past Infancy: Fact Sheet," Kelly Bonyata, KellyMom, last modified July 26, 2011, http://kellymom.com/ages/older-infant/ebf-benefits/.

28. Ibid.

29. Ibid.

30. "Breastfeeding Past Infancy: Fact Sheet," Kelly Bonyata, KellyMom, last modified July 26, 2011, http://kellymom.com/ages/older-infant/ebf-benefits/.

31. "How Much Money Does Breastfeeding Really Save?," Trent Hamm, The Simple Dollar, last modified December 10, 2013, http://www.thesimpledollar.com/how-much-money-does-breastfeeding-really-save/.

32. "Tandem Nursing," Breastfeeding Mother-to-Mother, last updated March 9, 2008, http://breastfeedingbasics.info/tandem-nursing.

33. "Breastfeeding, Family Physicians Supporting (Position Paper)," Policies, American Academy of Family Physicians, accessed May 26, 2014, http://www.aafp.org/about/policies/all/breastfeeding-support.html.

34. "Breastfeeding Tandem," Breastfeeding-Magazine.com, accessed May 26, 2014, http://www.breastfeeding-magazine.com/breastfeeding-tandem.html.

Chapter 11

1. I learned this technique in my natural birthing class. Closing my eyes and focusing on my breathing really helped the contractions

feel a lot shorter. I would breathe slowly—in through my nose and out through my mouth.

2. A doula is a woman that helps you through birth and typically performs pain management techniques to help ease contractions. She supports you and the family.

3. As the baby descends he or she is pushing some of your organs and clearing the path.

4. Nell Lake, "Labor, Interrupted," *Harvard Magazine*, November/December 2012, http://harvardmagazine.com/2012/11/labor-interrupted.

5. "Midwifery Model," About Midwives, Midwives Alliance of North America, accessed April 2, 2014, http://mana.org/about-midwives/midwifery-model.

6. Ibid.

7. Nell Lake, "Labor, Interrupted," *Harvard Magazine*, November/December 2012, http://harvardmagazine.com/2012/11/labor-interrupted.

8. Ibid.

9. Ibid.

Dr. Osborne holds a BA in Biology from Transylvania University, a MSN in Midwifery from Vanderbilt School of Nursing, and a MS and SD in maternal and child health from Harvard School of Public Health.

10. Ibid.

11. Ibid.

12. *The Business of Being Born*, directed by Abby Epstein (Red Envelope Entertainment, 2008), Netflix.

13. Mary Brophy Marcus, "Read The Labels, Because 'All Drugs Have Side Effects'," *USA Today*, August 3, 2011, http://usatoday30.usatoday.com/LIFE/usaedition/2011-08-04-Overthecounter-drug-dangers--_ST_U.htm.

14. Nell Lake, "Labor, Interrupted," *Harvard Magazine*, November/December 2012, http://harvardmagazine.com/2012/11/labor-interrupted.

15. "Pitocin FAQ," Childbirth.org, accessed April, 2, 2014, http://www.childbirth.org/articles/pit.html.

16. Nell Lake, "Labor, Interrupted," *Harvard Magazine*, November/December 2012, http://harvardmagazine.com/2012/11/labor-interrupted.

17. Ibid.

18. *The Business of Being Born*, directed by Abby Epstein (Red Envelope Entertainment, 2008), Netflix.

19. "Hormones In Labour & Birth - How Your Body Helps You," Sarah J. Buckley, BellyBelly.com.au, last modified March 2005. http://www.bellybelly.com.au/birth/ecstatic-birth-natures-hormonal-blueprint-for-labor#.VH40_fnF_a8.

20. T. K. Abboud, E. Sarkis, T. T. Hung, S. S. Khoo, L. Varakian, E. Henriksen, R. Noueihed, U. Goebelsmann, and Brett B. Gutsche, "Effects of Epidural Anesthesia During Labor on Maternal Plasma Beta-Endorphin Levels," *Obstetric Anesthesia Digest* 3, no. 4 (1983): 106, doi:10.1097/00132582-198312000-00006.

21. Ina May Gaskin, *Ina May's Guide to Childbirth* (New York: Bantam Books, 2003).

22. "The Importance of Skin to Skin Contact," International Breastfeeding Centre, accessed April, 2, 2014, http://www.nbci.ca/index.php?option=com_content&view=article&id=82:theimportance-of-skin-to-skin-contact-&catid=5:information&Itemid=17.

23. Ksenia Bystrova, Valentina Ivanova, Maigun Edhborg, Ann-Sofi Matthiesen, Anna-Berit Ransjö-Arvidson, Rifkat Mukhamedrakhimov, Kerstin Uvnäs-Moberg, and Ann-Marie Widström, "Early Contact Versus Separation: Effects on Mother-Infant Interaction One Year Later," *Birth* 36, no. 2 (2009): 97-109, doi:10.1111/j.1523-536X.2009.00307.x.

24. Ibid.

25. "The Importance of Skin to Skin Contact," International Breastfeeding Centre, April 2, 2014, http://www.nbci.ca/index.php?option=com_content&view=article&id=82:theimportance-of-skin-to-skin-contact-&catid=5:information&Itemid=17.

26. Marian F. MacDorman, T. J. Mathews, and Eugene Declercq, "NCHS Data Brief: Home Births in the United States, 1990-2009," Centers for Disease Control and Prevention, last modified January 26, 2012, http://www.cdc.gov/nchs/data/databriefs/db84.htm.

27. "Vaginal Delivery," Healthcare Bluebook, accessed April, 2, 2014, https://www.healthcarebluebook.com/page_ProcedureDetails.aspx?id=108&dataset=MD&g=Vaginal+Delivery.

28. "Cesarean Section," HealthCare Bluebook, accessed April 2, 2014, https://www.healthcarebluebook.com/page_ProcedureDetails.aspx?id=107&dataset=md&g=Cesarean+Section.

29. "The Benefits of a Vaginal Delivery," Danielle Buffardi, Pregnancy Blog, American Pregnancy Association, last modified February 03, 2012, http://www.americanpregnancy.org/pregnancyblog/2012/02/benefits-of-a-vaginal-birth/.

30. "Risks of a Cesarean Procedure," American Pregnancy Association, last modified January 2014, http://americanpregnancy.org/labor-and-birth/cesarean-risks/.

31. L. O. Lawani, O. B. Anozie, P. O. Ezeonu, and C. A. Iyoke, "Comparison of Outcomes Between Operative Vaginal Deliveries and Spontaneous Vaginal Deliveries in Southeast Nigeria," *International Journal of Gynecology and Obstetrics* 125, no. 3 (June 2014): 206-209, doi:10.1016/j.ijgo.2013.11.018.

32. Nell Lake, "Labor, Interrupted," *Harvard Magazine*, November/December 2012, http://harvardmagazine.com/2012/11/labor-interrupted.

33. Elizabeth A. Dunn and Colm O'Herlihy, "Comparison of Maternal Satisfaction Following Vaginal Delivery After Caesarean Section and Caesarean Section After Previous Vaginal Delivery," *European Journal of Obstetrics & Gynecology and Reproductive Biology* 121, no. 1 (2005): 56-60, doi:10.1016/j.ejogrb.2004.11.010.

34. Joanne Sullivan Marut and Ramona T. Mercer, "Comparison of Primiparas' Perceptions of Vaginal and Cesarean Births," *Nursing Research* 28, no. 5 (1979): 260-66.

35. Vincenzo Zanardo, Giorgia Svegliado, Francesco Cavallin, Arturo Giustardi, Erich Cosmi, Pietro Litta, and Daniele Trevisanuto, "Elective Cesarean Delivery: Does It Have a Negative Effect on Breastfeeding?," *Birth* 37, no. 4 (2010): 275-79, doi:10.1111/j.1523-536X.2010.00421.x.

36. Ibid.

37. E. L. Ryding, K. Wijma, and B. Wijma, "Psychological Impact of Emergency Cesarean Section In Comparison With Elective Cesarean Section, Instrumental and Normal Vaginal Delivery," *Journal of Psychosomatic Obstetrics & Gynecology* 19, no. 3 (1998): 135-44, doi:10.3109/01674829809025691.

38. "Childbirth," HMHB.org, accessed April 2, 2014, http://www.hmhb.org/virtual-library/interviews-with-experts/cesarean-section-c-section/.

E. L. Ryding, K. Wijma, and B. Wijma, "Psychological Impact of Emergency Cesarean Section In Comparison With

Elective Cesarean Section, Instrumental and Normal Vaginal Delivery," *Journal of Psychosomatic Obstetrics & Gynecology* 19, no. 3 (1998): 135-44, doi:10.3109/01674829809025691.

39. "Childbirth," HMHB.org, accessed April 2, 2014, http://www.hmhb.org/virtual-library/interviews-with-experts/cesarean-section-c-section/.

40. "The Benefits of a Vaginal Delivery," Danielle Buffardi, Pregnancy Blog, American Pregnancy Association, last modified February 03, 2012, http://www.americanpregnancy.org/pregnancyblog/2012/02/benefits-of-a-vaginal-birth/.

41. "Breastfeeding After a Cesarean," Anne Smith, Breastfeeding Basics, last modified September 2013, http://www.breastfeedingbasics.com/articles/breastfeeding-after-a-cesarean.

42. Nell Lake, "Labor, Interrupted," *Harvard Magazine*, November/December 2012, http://harvardmagazine.com/2012/11/labor-interrupted.

43. "Childbirth," HMHB.org, accessed April 2, 2014, http://www.hmhb.org/virtual-library/interviews-with-experts/cesarean-section-c-section/.

Chapter 12

1. "Kate's Unabashed Baby Belly Busts the Last Taboo of Pregnancy," Tom Sykes, The Daily Beast, last modified July 24, 2013, http://www.thedailybeast.com/articles/2013/07/24/kate-s-unabashed-baby-belly-busts-the-last-taboo-of-pregnancy.html.

2. "Study: Fish Oil May Prevent Symptoms of Postpartum Depression," Alice Park, Time.com, last modified April 12, 2011, http://healthland.time.com/2011/04/12/study-fish-oil-may-prevent-symptoms-of-postpartum-depression/.

3. "The Truth About Your Body After Baby," Aryen Jackson-Cannady, Fitness Magazine, accessed July, 1, 2014, http://www.fitness-magazine.com/weight-loss/baby/your-body-after-baby/?page=2.

Chapter 13

1. Brooke Fraser, "Hosanna," *All of the Above*, Hillsong Music Australia, compact disc, 2007.

Bonus Chapter

1. "Pesticides and Food: Why Children May Be Especially Sensitive to Pesticides," Pesticides: Health and Safety, EPA, last modified August 4, 2014, http://www.epa.gov/pesticides/food/pest.htm.

2. "Even Babies Need Exercise," John Casey, Health & Baby, WebMD, accessed April 14, 2014, http://www.webmd.com/parenting/baby/features/even-babies-need-exercise.

3. "The Case for Healthy Bowels: The Vital Connection Between Your Gut and Your Health," Mercola.com, last modified April 18, 2009, http://articles.mercola.com/sites/articles/archive/2009/04/18/probiotics-the-case-for-healthy-bowels.aspx.

4. "What Are Nambudripad's Allergy Elimination Techniques?," NAET Patients, accessed April 14, 2014, http://www.naet.com/Patients/whatsnaet.aspx.

5. Heinz F. Eichenwald, "Fever and Antipyresis," *Bulletin of the World Health Organization* 81, no.5 (2003): 372-374, doi: 10.1590/S0042-96862003000500012.

6. T. Vardam, L. Zhou, M. Appenheimer, Q. Chen, W. Wang, H. Baumann, and S. Evans, "Regulation of a Lymphocyte–Endothelial–IL-6 Trans-Signaling Axis By Fever-Range Thermal Stress: Hot Spot of Immune Surveillance," *Cytokine* 39, no. 1 (2007): 84-96, doi:10.1016/j.cyto.2007.07.184.

7. Baris E. Dayanc, Sarah H. Beachy, Julie R. Ostberg, and Elizabeth A. Repasky, "Dissecting the Role of Hyperthermia In Natural Killer Cell Mediated Anti-Tumor Responses," *International Journal of Hyperthermia* 24, no. 1 (2008): 41-56, doi:10.1080/02656730701858297.

8. Arianna Yanes, "Acetaminophen in Pregnancy Linked To 'ADHD-Like Behaviors'" *The Chart* (blog), CNN, February 24, 2014, http://thechart.blogs.cnn.com/2014/02/24/acetaminophen-in-pregnancy-linked-to-adhd-like-behaviors/.

9. "Baby Acetaminophen Tied to Asthma," Daniel J. DeNoon, Asthma Health Center, WebMD, last modified September 18, 2008, http://www.webmd.com/asthma/news/20080918/baby_acetaminophen_tied_to_asthma.

10. M. J. Kluger, "Is Fever Beneficial?," *Yale Journal of Biology and Medicine* 59, no. 2 (March/April 1986): 89-95.

Carl I. Schulman, Nicholas Namias, James Doherty, Ronald J. Manning, Pamela Li, Ahmed Elhaddad, David Lasko, Jose Amortegui, Christopher J. Dy, Lucie Dlugasch, Gio Baracco, and Stephen M. Cohn, "The Effect of Antipyretic Therapy Upon Outcomes In Critically Ill Patients: A Randomized, Prospective Study," *Surgical Infections* 6, no. 4 (2005): 369-75, doi:10.1089/sur.2005.6.369.

Su Fuhong, Nam Duc Nguyen, Wang Zhen, Peter Rogiers, and Jean-Louis Vincent, "Fever

Control in Septic Shock: Beneficial or Harmful?," *CHEST Journal* 124, no. 4 (2003), doi:10.1378/chest.124.4_MeetingAbstracts.225S-b.

11. "Febrile Seizures," MedlinePlus, last modified February 26, 2014, http://www.nlm.nih.gov/medlineplus/ency/article/000980.htm.

12. Aaron Rossi, "Fever-It's No Sweat," *A Health Philosophy* (blog), January 23, 2012, http://draaronrossi.blogspot.com/search/label/Fever.

13. Elaine Wirrell and Troy Turner, "Parental Anxiety and Family Disruption Following a First Febrile Seizure in Childhood," *Pediatrics & Child Health* 6, no. 3 (2001): 139-143.

14. "Fever," MedlinePlus, last modified February 1, 2012, http://www.nlm.nih.gov/medlineplus/ency/article/003090.htm.

15. Aaron Rossi, "Fever-It's No Sweat," *A Health Philosophy* (blog), January 23, 2012, http://draaronrossi.blogspot.com/search/label/Fever.

16. "How Long Can We Survive Without Food Or Water?," Canada, CBCnews, last modified May 09, 2011, http://www.cbc.ca/news/canada/how-long-can-we-survive-without-food-or-water-1.1000898.

17. "What Is Colorpuncture?," Colorpuncture.com, accessed April, 14, 2014, http://www.colorpuncture.com/whatis.html.

18. "Med Surg CH 16 Fluid & Electrolytes-Lab Values," Quizlet, accessed December 03, 2014, http://quizlet.com/21599243/med-surg-ch-16-fluid-electrolytes-lab-values-flash-cards/.

19. Dawn Throne, "Should We Fear Fever?," *Fountain of Healthy News*, September 2006, http://www.fountainofhealth.com/newsletters/2006/sep2006.php.

20. "Febrile Seizures Fact Sheet," National Institute of Neurological Disorders and Stroke, last modified April 16, 2014, http://www.ninds.nih.gov/disorders/febrile_seizures/detail_febrile_seizures.htm.

21. "Febrile Seizures: Guideline for the Neurodiagnostic Evaluation of the Child With a Simple Febrile Seizure," *Pediatrics* 127, no. 2 (2011): 389-94, doi:10.1542/peds.2010-3318.

22. "Febrile Seizures," MedlinePlus, last modified February 26, 2014, http://www.nlm.nih.gov/medlineplus/ency/article/000980.htm.

Barton D. Schmitt, *Your Child's Health: The Parents' One-Stop Reference Guide to Symptoms, Emergencies, Common Illnesses, Behavior Problems, Healthy Development*, 2nd revision (New York: Bantam Books, 2005), 41.

23. Robert Frost, "The Road Not Taken," line 20.

Index

A

acetaminophen 12
acne 84, 150
ADHD 13, 97
adoption 155, 157, 159
affordable 6, 32, 34, 46, 64, 68, 84
    save 26–27, 34, 63, 84, 112, 119, 174
alcohol 7, 11, 81
allergies 3, 28, 58–59, 62, 170
almond oil 80, 82
amniotic fluid 30, 87, 97, 118–119, 133, 144, 147
anemia 9, 81
anesthesia 127, 137, 142–143
asthma xiii, xiv, 13, 55, 56, 58–59, 76, 144, 152, 170

B

baby blues 90, 149
baby carrier 150
back pain xiv, 38, 68, 70, 71, 76–77, 149
baths 82, 173
beauty products 6, 85
belly 6, 18, 38, 51, 70, 80, 83, 87, 89, 94, 147
BioElectrical Impedance Measurement (BIM) 59–60
birth control 1, 3, 11
birthing center 23, 129, 131, 134, 142, 144–145
birth plan xx, xxi, 73, 104, 117, 123–124, 130–131, 145
BMI 5
bonding with your baby 85, 101
bouncing back xxi, 147–148, 151–152
Braxton-Hicks xix, 76, 87
breastfeeding v, xv, 8, 9, 14, 26, 32, 34, 75, 90, 103–106, 108–115, 129, 136, 140–145, 149, 151–152, 170
breasts 6, 80, 87, 104, 108, 110, 114
breathing through contractions 120, 122, 130
breech 73–74, 127–128, 137, 144
burpees 37–38, 151

C

caffeine 7, 11, 19, 46
calcium 8, 14, 63, 82, 109, 171, 173
celiac disease 28, 183
cesarean 126–127, 138, 143–145
changes by trimester 86
childbirth i, v, xi, 38–39, 52, 72, 82, 101, 119, 125, 129, 136–137, 139, 148
chiropractic/chiropractor xiv, xvi, xxi, 2, 3, 51, 67–77, 79, 95, 98, 107, 120, 127, 135, 137, 149, 166–167, 170
chlorophyll 60, 61, 63
church 55, 94–95, 155–157, 159, 166, 179
coconut oil 6, 8, 19, 27, 29, 30–31, 58, 80, 82, 84, 105, 171, 174
coffee enemas 4, 178
colostrum 87, 104
communication 33, 98, 129–130
compresses 75, 83, 123
conception xvi, xxi, 2–6, 8–9, 15, 148
constipation 25–26, 38, 61, 63, 87
contractions xix, 23, 26, 75–77, 84, 87, 118–122, 129–131, 134–139, 141, 144
cord blood banking 141
cortisol 39, 96–98
cramps 28, 120, 139
cravings 17–18, 23, 27
c-section 40, 76, 124–130, 136, 138, 142–144

D

delivery xix, 18, 39, 41, 50, 68, 83, 114, 117, 125, 127–128, 137, 140–145, 148, 155
detox 2–4, 7–8, 11, 178
dopplers 86, 88, 128
drugs xiii, 12, 130, 136–138, 172

E

eggs 7, 27, 29
energy 2, 4, 6, 8, 14, 18, 25, 28, 37, 46–48, 50–51, 60, 67, 69–71, 76, 90, 117, 119, 120, 122, 133, 148–149, 167, 169–170
Environmental Working Group (EWG) 13, 25, 32, 34, 81
epidural 124, 127, 130, 135–139
epilepsy 13, 167, 174
episiotomy 83, 89, 133, 138
exercise 5–6, 37–41, 72, 79, 83, 85, 98, 131, 149, 168–169, 178
  Insanity 38, 41
eye mask 51

F

facials 83
faith 94, 96, 99, 156, 167
family vi, xiii, xiv, xvi, xxi, 4, 27, 34, 38, 41, 48, 68, 72, 94, 97, 120, 131, 135–137, 148, 157, 159, 168, 170, 175, 178
fast food 6, 7, 23–24
fasting 7
fatigue 13, 38, 47, 49, 87, 89
feeling good 3–4
fertility 1, 2, 11, 13, 112, 143
first foods 115, 168
folate 7, 9–10, 61

G

genetically modified foods (GMOs) 21, 25, 30, 31, 32
gestational diabetes 38, 112
ginger 26, 61, 62

gingivitis 6, 82
glucose 30, 125
gluten-free 19, 28, 29

H

headaches 12, 26, 67, 87, 96
heal 67, 69, 71, 166, 172
health issues 2, 13, 149
healthy baby vi, 40, 101, 165–168
hemorrhage 143–144
hemorrhoids 87
home birth i, xix, 73, 77, 99, 130, 134, 142, 144–145
hospital birth 125, 130–131, 134, 142
how to buy organic 22, 29

I

immune system 3, 7, 24, 27–28, 47–48, 58–60, 71, 96–97, 166, 169–172
induction 40
insurance 2, 56, 64
iridology 2, 57, 59
iron 14, 19, 26, 60–62
irregular contractions 76, 87
IVF 2

J

juicing 4, 24–26

K

Kegels 83, 148

L

labor xi, xvi, xix–xx, 22–24, 27, 38–41, 50, 72, 74–77, 82–84, 89, 97, 101, 110, 117–129, 131, 133, 135–141, 144, 148, 152
linea nigra 87
looking good 6

M

manicure 6, 83–84, 150
massage 83–84, 90, 148
microwaving 10
midwife xvi, xxi, xix, 23, 27, 38–39, 73, 76, 98, 106–107, 118–119, 124–129, 131, 133–135, 139, 140, 142, 144–145
mortality rate 111, 125, 134
muscle test 57, 75

N

napping 45–52, 72, 98, 117, 169
natural oils 6, 80–82, 84
naturopathic treatment xiii, 1–2, 55, 57, 59–60, 98
nausea 87, 89, 129
nursing 103–108, 110, 112, 114, 140, 168, 171
nutrition xxi, 5, 7, 10, 18, 23, 32, 79, 109, 142, 149, 168, 170
  nutrients to consume 7

O

organic 6, 8, 14, 19, 21, 22, 25, 27, 29–34, 80, 81, 150, 168, 174
oxytocin 89, 139, 141

P

pain xiv, 1, 38–39, 51, 67–72, 75–77, 87, 89, 131, 133–136, 138–139, 143, 149, 155, 177
pain-free delivery 155
parabens 14, 81
PCOS 1
pedicures 83, 150
pelvis 41, 74–76, 137
pillows 51, 137
pitocin 138, 144
placenta 9, 11, 97, 128, 141, 143, 145, 147
PLU codes 33–34
postpartum 40, 128, 143–144, 147, 149–150, 177
prayer 99–100
preeclampsia 8–9
pregnancy i, v–vi, xi, xiv, xix–xxii, 2–9, 11–12, 17–18, 22–27, 29, 34, 37–41, 47, 50–51, 57–61, 63–64, 68, 71–74, 76–77, 79, 82–90, 95–98, 100–101, 104, 109, 112, 114, 117–118, 123–126, 129, 131, 133, 136, 141, 143, 145, 147–151, 155, 177–179
pregnancy diet 22, 24, 60–61
preheating ix, xxi, 1–3, 6–7, 9–12, 15, 67, 80
prenatal 2, 8–9, 23, 61, 63, 71, 83, 86, 88, 97, 107, 109, 115, 124–125, 129
prenatal stress 97
preparing for conception xxi
pressure 13, 26–27, 67, 72, 74–75, 87, 96–97, 110, 120, 122, 129, 144–145, 172
protein 7, 10, 14, 19, 27–28, 60–63, 109
pubic bone adjustment 76

R

radiation 10, 68, 86, 88
relaxin 38
respiratory problems 3, 111, 144

rest 5, 45–51, 70, 77, 98, 117–119, 147–148, 156, 169, 175
restless legs 8
rGBH 31–32

S

smoking 12
sensation 119, 120, 122, 133, 138–139, 148
sex during pregnancy 79, 88–90, 157
shea butter 84, 174
skin care 6
sleep 4, 13, 38, 46–49, 50–51, 96, 98, 104, 114, 119, 137, 168
sleeping position 50, 87
smoothies 19, 63, 84, 149
soaps 14, 80–81, 84
soy 27, 30–32, 61–62
spinal cord 2, 9, 69–70
squats 38, 41, 83
stress 38–40, 47–48, 51, 70–72, 93–99, 101, 133, 143, 145, 150, 168
   stress remedies 98
stretching 6, 41, 82, 122
stretch marks 6, 80, 87, 150
sunscreen 84
symptoms 3, 12, 38, 76, 86–87, 97–98, 129, 175

T

teeth and gums 6
the business of being born 73, 129, 139
the flu shot 14–15
things to avoid 3, 10
toothpaste 13, 82, 84

trimesters 3, 6, 9, 41, 51, 57, 59, 63, 79, 82–83, 86–89, 93, 97
true health vi, xiii–xiv, xvi, xxi-xxii, 21, 57, 179

U

ultrasound 9, 68, 75, 86, 88, 125, 128
uterus 47, 74, 89, 126, 138, 141, 144, 147, 149

V

vaginal birth 39, 125–126, 142–143
Vitamin D 8, 63, 82, 109, 150, 169
vitamin E 8

W

water i, xix–xx, 7, 12, 13, 25–27, 40, 58, 60–63, 75, 82–84, 112, 118–123, 128, 131, 133–136, 139, 141, 148, 151, 166, 171–173
waxing 84
webster technique 73–74
weight xiii, xxi, 4–5, 23–24, 26, 30, 40, 42, 87, 96–97, 106, 109, 112, 147–148, 150, 178
what to eat 3, 6
white blood cells 11, 173
whole foods 7, 19, 24
working out 37–38, 40–42, 85, 117, 148
World Health Organization (WHO) 106, 125
worrying 98–99

X

x-rays 6, 68, 75, 88

Photo Credits

Back cover	Ginelle Lago // GMNArtistic.com
Page xii	Alex Herrera Photography
Page xxiii	Ginelle Lago // GMNArtistic.com
Page 4	Chris Sosa Photography
Page 22	Chris Sosa Photography
Page 23	Chris Sosa Photography
Page 24	Omar Saavedra
Page 27	Chris Sosa Photography
Page 42	Chris Sosa Photography
Page 53	Chris Sosa Photography
Page 56	Unknown
Page 80	Chris Sosa Photography
Page 91	Alex Herrera Photography
Page 100	Chris Sosa Photography
Page 105	Alex Herrera Photography
Page 121	Chris Sosa Photography
Page 132	Chris Sosa Photography
Page 153	Chris Sosa Photography
Page 161	Chris Sosa Photography
Page 162	Chris Sosa Photography
Page 163	Chris Sosa Photography
Page 176	Augusto Marquez
Page 179	Ginelle Lago // GMNArtistic.com
Page 180	Chris Sosa Photography

www.ingramcontent.com/pod-product-compliance
Lightning Source LLC
Chambersburg PA
CBHW041247240426
43669CB00026B/2994